Infecting the Ancient Mesopotamian Cosmos

Die babylonisch-assyrische Medizin in Texten und Untersuchungen

---

Begründet von Franz Köcher

Herausgegeben von
Nils P. Heeßel und Marten Stol

Band 14

Infecting the Ancient Mesopotamian Cosmos

Epidemics and the Transmission of Disease in Assyria and Babylonia

Edited by
Troels P. Arbøll

DE GRUYTER

ISBN 978-3-11-223861-5
ISBN 978-3-11-223862-2 (PDF)
ISBN 978-3-11-223863-9 (EPUB)
DOI https://doi.org/10.1515/9783112238622

Library of Congress Control Number: 2026933451

Bibliographic information published by the Deutsche Nationalbibliothek
The Deutsche Nationalbibliothek lists this publication in the Deutsche Nationalbibliografie; detailed bibliographic data are available on the Internet at http://dnb.dnb.de.

De Gruyter and Walter de Gruyter GmbH are part of De Gruyter Brill.
www.degruyterbrill.com

Questions about General Product Safety Regulation:
productsafety@degruyterbrill.com

Cover illustration: Amulet with an extract from the Erra Epic,
intended to ward off plague and evil (BM 118998). © The Trustees of the British Museum.

Acknowledgements

This volume has its origins in the conference *Infecting the Ancient Mesopotamian Cosmos*, which took place over two days from the 29th to the 30th of April 2022 at Wolfson College in the Leonard Wolfson Auditorium at the University of Oxford. It was held at a unique moment in time, just as the world was beginning to open up once again following the COVID-19 pandemic. For many of us, it was the first opportunity to gather in person, and what better theme for this occasion than the study of some of history's earliest recorded epidemics, as described in cuneiform sources from ancient Mesopotamia? Rarely had ancient Near Eastern studies felt more contemporary.

The aim of the conference was to explore the ancient conceptions and effects of transmissible diseases through the study of cuneiform texts. Specifically, the gathering addressed how people in ancient Mesopotamia envisioned and described widespread diseases, how such afflictions were believed to spread throughout society, and how people attempted to counter such afflictions through pragmatic and magico-medical means. In a larger perspective, the meeting explored inauspicious portents and astrology in relation to transmissible illnesses, and how diseases were believed to spread between animals, humans, and households. Finally, the conference considered how communicable diseases were situated in a larger cosmic setting, and in which ways mythological or literary narratives provided etiologies for understanding what it meant to be ill. This volume bears witness to those efforts, though unfortunately, not all participants were able to submit a written version of their papers. Furthermore, I tried to incorporate at least one paper addressing the Hittite perspective on communicable diseases, though this proved impossible at the time.

The conference was organized as part of my Junior Research Fellowship at Linacre College, University of Oxford, and I am grateful to the funding bodies that strongly supported the conference and made it possible, namely the Carlsberg Foundation, the British Institute for the Study of Iraq, and the General Fund for Assyriology at Wolfson College, Oxford. The final editing of this volume was conducted during my assistant professorship at the Department of Cross-Cultural and Regional Studies, University of Copenhagen, generously funded by the Edubba Foundation.

I extend my sincere thanks to all the speakers who contributed their expertise and insights by kindly accepting my invitation to present at the gathering, namely Annie Attia, Barbara Böck, Eckart Frahm, Nils Heeßel, Adam Howe, Marta Iommelli, Ulla Koch, and JoAnn Scurlock. Their presentations and discussions provided the foundation for this volume. Given the circumstances of the time, I am thankful to the speakers who were unable to travel and therefore presented over Zoom. Robert Arnott, who had supported my preparation, had planned to present a promising paper on disease along trade routes between Mesopotamia, the Gulf, and the Indus Civilization. Sadly, he fell ill some days before the conference and was unable to attend. I was saddened to read about his passing in 2024.

Throughout my preparations, and during the conference, Jacob Dahl provided unwavering support and encouragement, and it is a pleasure to express my gratitude here. I am indebted to Moudhy Al-Rashid, Nils Heeßel, Ulla Koch, and Kathryn Stevens for kindly agreeing to participate as session chairs, and I am grateful for their contributions to the discussions. Moudhy Al-Rashid deserves special recognition for her thoughtful inputs throughout the planning process and for raising many important topics that were included in the final discussion. Furthermore, I am thankful to William Skelton who volunteered to assist with practicalities during the gathering. I am equally indebted to all the participants in the audience for their constructive comments and contributions during the discussions. Stephanie Dalley deserves special recognition for sharing numerous valuable insights.

For his careful and constructive peer review, I extend my warmest thanks to the series editor Marten Stol, whose feedback greatly strengthened this volume. I would also like to express my gratitude to Albrecht Döhnert, the editorial director responsible for the BAM series, who kindly facilitated the publication of this monograph. Furthermore, I am truly grateful to Antonia Pohl for checking and preparing the manuscript for publication. The book itself follows the bibliographical style and formatting of previous volumes in the BAM series, though a few editorial choices may differ slightly from past conventions.

It is my hope that the collective contributions in this volume will serve as a significant step towards establishing a renewed foundation for the study of epidemics in ancient Mesopotamia. This field of research holds a substantial potential for Assyriological, archaeological and interdisciplinary research, which can greatly enrich and shape future scholarship on the conceptualization, understanding, and impact of widespread disease in the ancient world.

T.P.A.
Copenhagen, February 2025

Contents

List of Abbreviations

AbB 2	R. Frankena, *Briefe aus dem British Museum (LIH und CT 2–33)* (1966)
ADD	C. H. W. Johns, *Assyrian Deeds and Documents Recording the Transfer of Property . . . Chiefly of the 7th Century B.C., Volume 1* (1898)
AHw	W. von Soden, *Akkadisches Handwörterbuch, vol. 1–3* (1965–1981)
AMC	Assur Medical Catalogue, see BAM 9
ARM 3	J. R. Kupper, *Correspondance de Kibri-Dagan*, Archives Royales de Mari 3 (1950)
ARM 5	G. Dossin, *Correspondance de Iasmaḫ-Addu*, Archives Royales de Mari 5 (1952)
ARM 10	G. Dossin and A. Finet, *Correspondance féminine*, Archives Royales de Mari 10 (1978)
ARM 13	G. Dossin, J. Bottéro, M. Birot, M. Lurton Burke, J.-R. Kupper, and A. Finet, *Textes Divers*, Archives Royales de Mari 13 (1964)
ARM 14	M. Birot, *Lettres de Yaqqim-Addu gouverneur de Sagarâtum*, Archives Royales de Mari 14 (1974)
ARM 26/1	J.-M. Durand, *Archives Épistolaires de Mari 1/1,* Archives Royales de Mari 26/1 (1988)
ARM 27	M. Birot, *Correspondance des Gouverneurs de Qaṭṭunân*, Archives Royales de Mari 27 (1993)
ARM 33	J.-M. Durand, *Les premières années du roi Zimrî-Lîm de Mari*, Archives Royales de Mari 33 (2019)
BAM	F. Köcher, *Die babylonisch-assyrische Medizin in Texten und Untersuchungen, Volumes 1-6* (1963-80) / M. J. Geller, *Die babylonisch-assyrische Medizin in Texten und Untersuchungen, Volumes 7-8* (2005-16) / U. Steinert (ed.), *Die babylonisch-assyrische Medizin in Texten und Untersuchungen, Volume 9* (2018) / M. J. Geller and S. V. Panayotov, *Die babylonisch-assyrische Medizin in Texten und Untersuchungen, Volume 10* (2020) / J. C. Johnson and K. Simkó, *Die babylonisch-assyrische Medizin in Texten und Untersuchungen, Volume 11* (2024) / U. Steinert, *Die babylonisch-assyrische Medizin in Texten und Untersuchungen, Volume 12* (2026) / E. Schmidtchen, *Die babylonisch-assyrische Medizin in Texten und Untersuchungen, Volume 13* (2021)
CAD	A. L. Oppenheim, E. Reiner et al., *The Assyrian Dictionary of the Oriental Institute of the University of Chicago* (1956–2010)
CALPo	Comprehensive Aramaic Lexicon Project online <https://cal.huc.edu> (accessed 25/02/2024)
CTN 4	D. J. Wiseman and J. A. Black, *Literary Texts from the Temple of Nabû*, Cuneiform Texts from Nimrud 4 (1996)
CMAwR	T. Abusch and D. Schwemer, *Corpus of Mesopotamian Anti-Witchcraft Rituals. Volume 1*, Ancient Magic and Divination 8/1 (2011) / T. Abusch, D. Schwemer, M. Luukko, and G. van Buylaere, *Corpus of Mesopotamian Anti-Witchcraft Rituals. Volume 2*, Ancient Magic and Divination 8/2 (2016) / T. Abusch, D. Schwemer, M. Luukko, and G. van Buylaere, *Corpus of Mesopotamian Anti-Witchcraft Rituals. Volume 3*, Ancient Magic and Divination 8/3 (2020) / G. van Buylaere and M. Luukko, *Corpus of Mesopotamian Anti-Witchcraft Rituals Glossaries and Indices*, Ancient Magic and Divination 8/4 (2020)
DPS	R. Labat, *Traité akkadien de diagnostics et prognostics médicaux I–II*, Collection de Travaux de l'Académie Internationale d'Historie des Sciences 7 (1951) / N. P. Heeßel, *Babylonisch-assyrische Diagnostik*, Alter Orient und Altes Testament 43 (2000) / J.-A. Scurlock, *Sourcebook for Ancient Mesopotamian Medicine*, Writings from the Ancient World 36 (2014), 13–272 / see BAM 13 and SA.GIG
EA	W. Moran, *The Amarna Letters* (1992)
eBL	The "electronic Babylonian Library" Platform <https://www.ebl.lmu.de> (accessed 06/02/2025)
Ee	*Enuma eliš* (Babylonian creation myth)
ePSD2	The New Version of the Electronic Pennsylvania Sumerian Dictionary <http://oracc.museum.upenn.edu/epsd2/index.html> (accessed 07/12/2021)
eSAD	electronic Supplement to the Akkadian Dictionaries <https://www.gkr.uni-leipzig.de/altorientalisches-institut/forschung/supplement-to-the-akkadian-dictionaries> (accessed 25/02/2024).
FMA	J. Sasson, *From the Mari Archives: An Anthology of Old Babylonian Letters*. State College: (2017).
LAPO 17	J.-M. Durand, *Les documents épistolaires du palais de Mari II*, Littératures Anciennes du Proche-Orient 17 (1998)
LAPO 18	J. M. Durand, *Les documents épistolaires du palais de Mari III*, Littératures Anciennes du Proche-Orient 18 (2000)
KUB	*Keilschrifturkunden aus Boghazköi*
Ludlul	*Ludlul bēl nēmeqi*; A. Annus and A. Lenzi, *Ludlul bēl nēmeqi*, State Archives of Assyria Cuneiform Texts 7 (2010) / T. Oshima, *Babylonian Poems of Pious Sufferers*, Orientalische Religionen in der Antike 14 (2014), 78–114 / A. Lenzi, *Suffering in Babylon*, Orbis Biblicus et Orientalis 300 (2023), 64–94
Lugal-e	J. van Dijk, *Lugal UD ME-LÁM-bi NIR.GÁL: Le récit épique et didactique des Travaux de Ninurta, du Déluge et de la Nouvelle Création. Tome II* (1983) / S. Seminara, *La versione accadica del Lugal-e*, Materiali per il Vocabolario Sumerico 8 (2001)
Maqlû	T. Abusch, *The Witchcraft series Maqlû*, Writings from the Ancient World 37 (2015) / D. Schwemer, *The Anti-Witchcraft Ritual Maqlû: The Cuneiform Sources of a Magic Ceremony from Ancient Mesopotamia* (2017)
MSL 2	B. Landsberger, *Die Serie Ur-e-a = nâqu*, Materialien zum Sumerischen Lexikon 2 (1951)
MSL 8/1	B. Landsberger, *The Fauna of Ancient Mesopotamia. First Part*, Materialien zum Sumerischen Lexikon 8/1 (1960)
NARGD	J. N. Postgate, *Neo-Assyrian Royal Grants and Decrees*, Studia Pohl (Series Maior) 1 (1969)
Obv.	Obverse of a manuscript
ORACC	The Open Richly Annotated Cuneiform Corpus online <https://oracc.museum.upenn.edu> (accessed 06/02/2025)
Pausanius	Pausanius' Description of Greece online at ToposText <https://topostext.org/work/213> (accessed 30/01/2025)
PEI	The Poem of Erra and Išum, see L. Cagni, *L'Epopea di Erra*, Studi Semitici 34 (1969)
Rev.	Reverse of a manuscript
RIMA 1	A. K. Grayson, *Assyrian Rulers of the Third and Second Millennia BC (to 1115 BC)*, The Royal Inscriptions of Mesopotamia Assyrian Periods Volume 1 (1987)

 | https://doi.org/10.1515/9783112238622-204

RIMA 2	A. K. Grayson, *Assyrian Rulers of the Early First Millennium BC I (114–859 BC)*, The Royal Inscriptions of Mesopotamia Assyrian Periods Volume 2 (1991)
RIMB 2	G. Frame, *Rulers of Babylonia From the Second Dynasty of Isin to the End of Assyrian Domination (1157–612 BC)*, The Royal Inscriptions of Mesopotamia Babylonian Periods Volume 2 (1995)
RINAPo	The Royal Inscriptions of Assyria online <https://oracc.museum.upenn.edu/riao/> (accessed 06/02/2025)
SAA 2	S. Parpola and K. Watanabe, *Neo-Assyrian Treaties and Loyalty Oath*, State Archives of Assyria 2 (1988)
SAA 3	A. Livingstone, *Court Poetry and Literary Miscellanea*, State Archives of Assyria 3 (1959)
SAA 8	H. Hunger, *Astrological reports to Assyrian kings*, State Archives of Assyria 8 (1992).
SAA 10	S. Parpola, *Letters from Assyrian and Babylonian Scholars*, State Archives of Assyria 10 (1993)
SAA 12	L. Kataja and R. Whiting, *Grants, Decrees and Gifts of the Neo-Assyrian Period*, State Archives of Assyria 12 (1995)
SAA 19	M. Luukko, *The Correspondence of Tiglath-Pileser III and Sargon II from Calah/Nimrud*, State Archives of Assyria 19 (2012).
SAAo	The State Archives of Assyria online <https://oracc.museum.upenn.edu/saao/> (accessed 06/02/2025)
SA.GIG	The diagnostic omen series Sa-gig/*Sakikkû* (The Diagnostic Handbook), see DPS
SpTU I	H. Hunger, *Spätbabylonische Texte aus Uruk, Teil 1* (1976)
StBoT	Studien zu den Boğazköy-Texten
Šurpu	E. Reiner, *Šurpu: A Collection of Sumerian and Akkadian Incantations* (1958)
UH	Udug-ḫul, see BAM 8
Ur$_5$-ra	The lexical list Ur$_5$/ḪAR-ra = *ḫubullu*
YOS	Yale Oriental Series. Babylonian Texts

For other abbreviations, see the Cuneiform Digital Library Initiative list of abbreviations <https://cdli.mpiwg-berlin.mpg.de/abbreviations> (accessed 08/02/2024).

Troels P. Arbøll

Introduction

We are a plague on earth . . .
Either we limit our population growth,
or the natural world will do it for us,
and the natural world is doing it
for us right now.
David Attenborough, 2013

Epidemics are like ebb and flow, they continuously come and go. In the long span of human prehistory, it is commonly assumed that infections with the potential to become widespread among humans have existed for millennia, and one of the earliest identified infectious diseases has been discovered in a 31,600 year old individual (Nielsen et al. 2021).[1] Yet, it is reasonable to presume that when people settled in the world's first metropolises, the spread of infections accelerated to a hitherto unknown degree due to the multitude of people living closely together. The somewhat hazy and urban beginning of epidemic history, probably occurring over several thousand years, coincided at some point with the advent of written history, heralded by the invention of the cuneiform script in ancient Mesopotamia around 3,200 BCE and in use until 80 CE. It is therefore not surprising that ancient Mesopotamia offers some of the first written sources conceptualizing ancient epidemics. Groups of people regularly suffered from identical medical symptoms, or a large number of deaths attributed to the same overall cause. A multitude of terms for such phenomena are known from cuneiform texts, and these words and phrases are often translated as plagues, pestilences, or epidemics, though the exact meaning of these terms are often not properly elucidated. This volume provides new perspectives on epidemics in ancient Mesopotamia by examining how people experienced and reacted to infections, specifically epidemic diseases, described in cuneiform sources from Assyria and Babylonia from the 3rd until the end of the 1st millennium BCE.

In recent years the world experienced a seemingly extraordinary event, as societies over the globe faced a worldwide pandemic caused by COVID-19. This catastrophic event tested people's ability to live under intense conditions, and a multitude of explanations for this phenomenon surfaced. Despite scientific warnings through the past decade foreshadowing the rise of a new pandemic, most humans had seemingly learned nothing from similar events in the past, as the situation caused by COVID-19 seemed new and unexpected to most. Considering the longevity of written history, one of the purposes of these proceedings is to ask: What are the sources for studying epidemics in cuneiform writing, constituting some of humanity's earliest written sources? And how did humans in ancient Mesopotamia experience, describe, and conceptualize widespread diseases, such as epidemics and pandemics? Naturally, the COVID-19 pandemic has spawned a host of new studied in most disciplines. And with this volume, it is the hope of the editor to make the topic have a renewed impact on Assyriology and the study of the ancient Near East as well, by focusing on transmissible diseases in ancient Iraq.

Throughout history, epidemics have had severe effects on populations and the societies people live in (Scheidel 2017: 314–342), and they continue to be a major influence on historical change (Snowden 2020: 2). Perhaps unsurprisingly, they often cause or coincide with stagnation of living standards, poor harvest yields, depletion of livestock, and famine (Scheidel 2017: 297–298). Or in the words of Garrett Hardin (1993: 260): "Nature's two great tools for population control are starvation and disease". It is therefore possible that catastrophes leading to human suffering were indistinguishable from one another, as people "could as easily be devastated by a disease that swept through their flocks or their grain fields as by a plague that menaced them directly" (Scott 2017: 98). In fact, it might even have been considered unimportant what caused such cases of death: starvation causing weakened states or ensuing sickness (Hardin 1993: 262). Yet, because epidemics are such terrifying phenomena they create a need for understanding (Rosenberg 1992: 294).

1 The exact point of origin for many epidemic diseases as well as their relationship to humans is often unclear (Nielsen et al. 2021). Note that the study by Nielsen et al. has not yet been peer reviewed. Remains of ancient DNA from epidemic diseases have been found for e.g. *Yersinia pestis* (ca. 5.000 years old, Rasmussen et al. 2015), Epstein-Barr virus (ca. 5.700 year old, Jensen et al. 2019: 3, 5), and smallpox (ca. Viking age, Mühlemann et al. 2020; cf. Duggan et al. 2016; Ferrari et al. 2020).

Troels P. Arbøll, University of Copenhagen

 | https://doi.org/10.1515/9783112238622-001

Epidemics affect societies at large by influencing physical suffering, social relations, societal institutions, and can result in moral crises and stigmatizing discourses, whereby they can overturn ways of living (Keck et al. 2019: 1, 3; Herring and Swedlund 2010: 18–19, 232). At the same time, they can be discussed as potential facilitators driving societal development forward in e.g. religion and intellectual history (Snowden 2020: 2). Epidemics are therefore not only illnesses but they are also disruptive forces facilitating change.

Human overpopulation may be a dominant force in the rise of epidemics diseases, in combination with a disruption in the balance between humans and nature (Spernovasilis et al. 2021). And humanity's impact on nature is a commonly researched topic these years, due to a rising interest in climate change and biodiversity loss (United Nations 2022). In relation to ancient studies, the editor of these proceedings called for a new research agenda in Assyriology in a recent article in order to reassess the impact of ancient invasions of foreign territories, agricultural changes, as well as imports and redistribution of flora and fauna on the emergence of new epidemic diseases and outlining the ancient conditions under which they thrive.[2]

The study of ancient epidemics contains a number of inherent issues. For example, research occasionally rely on retrospective diagnoses, correlating ancient illness concepts with modern diseases, though little is known of the symptomology of most ancient epidemics (see von Weiher 2000, pp. 48–49; Klengel 1999). Another fundamental problem concerns the definition and use of the word epidemic for a rather broad variety of primarily Akkadian terms (see below). And it is not always clear if specific words or concrete episodes in texts truly represent a pandemic, epidemic, or simply an infectious disease. In terms of terminology, this is an issue from our perspective regarding how to describe the ancient thoughts on the matter. Accordingly, it has been discussed – without definite answer – when a disease outbreak should be considered epidemic (Herring and Swedlund 2010: 18). Furthermore, the terms epidemic and pandemic are problematic in an ancient context, as they have connotations of a single defined medical cause in a modern context (Martin and Martin-Granel 2006: 976–980). From the perspective of ancient sources, much information is missing, and without these details, it is practically impossible to label an infectious disease as an epidemic in modern terms. Similarly, conceptualization and context are crucial when translating the ancient terms, and researchers must be aware how to phrase these problems when making evidence available outside of Assyriology, as binary translations may skew or simplify the evidence in the eyes of non-specialists. Though various concrete criteria for the use of the terms epidemic and pandemic could be established on social, cultural, or purely scientific grounds, the contributions in this volume generally employs the term, and associated expressions, to signify any kind of transmissible disease with the potential to spread widely and sometimes rapidly among humans and/or animals. In some cases, individual articles will note if specific nuances are added to the use of such modern terms.

Another problem relates to descriptions of the transmission of sickness and evils, as well as the role of physical and social contact.[3] How were such afflictions believed to be transmitted by people in ancient Mesopotamia? We often use the terms contagion and contamination in the scholarly literature, but do any of these capture how people in the ancient Near East believed ailments were transmitted? In an article from 2000, Vivian Nutton cautioned researchers that the term contagion carries a preconceived notion of physical contact in relation to disease transmission, although this may not necessarily reflect ancient beliefs. Still, contamination through physical contact is a universal cognitive mechanism based on the idea that "physical contact between the source and the target results in the transfer of some effect or quality (essence) from the source to the target" (Nemeroff and Rozin 2000: 3). In cognitive studies of magic, contagion may even be "metaphorically extended to cover instances of seeing and hearing" (Sørensen 2007: 103). Feder (2016: 100) advanced on these views in relation to the ancient Near East, and he saw the "perception of the spread of an invisible force or essence" as "tied to a reaction of disgust and often fear which is elicited by contact (or potential contact) with various sources of contamination, both physiological (such as waste matter, insects, and disease-infected entities) and social, motivated by personal contempt, moral disdain, or racial biases". Or in the words of Farber (2004: 124): "Through such contact, one 'bad apple' could rot the whole basket, or make a whole town ill" (see also Ermidoro 2020: 32; Feder 2016: 107). A similar problem involves the term zoonosis, meaning a sickness transmitted from an animal to a human (for Mesopotamia, see Arbøll 2021: 24–27 with further references). The emergence of transmissible diseases with the

2 Arbøll 2024: 26. For example, there is evidence that humans changed the landscape in the early Holocene in the Levant, which caused changes to local fauna (Yeomans et al. 2024). Such evidence, alongside which plants were cultivated in different periods, should also be considered in future studies.

3 In addition to the literature cited below, note the series of six articles on hygiene in the ancient Near East published in *KASKAL NS* 1 (2024).

ability to spread between animals and humans, so-called zoonotic diseases, is of central interest to modern researchers of epidemic history.

Nutton is justified in his critique of the primary focus on physical contact as the point of transmission in an ancient context, though an idea of contagion may be applicable to some aspects of Mesopotamian thought (see Arbøll 2021: 25–26). For example, deities or demons could "touch" (*lapātu*), "seize" (*ṣabātu*), and "hit" (*maḫāṣu*) the unfortunate when afflicting disease (Salin 2015). From a modern point of view, such descriptions are at an intersection between religion and medicine, though for people in ancient Mesopotamia the wording likely reflected reality, similar to being injured during a fight (see van der Toorn 1985: 68). Still, physical contact between persons or objects was not a prerequisite for transferring evil, and some diseases considered transmissible in the ancient Middle East were likely not communicable from a modern perspective (e.g. *bennu*-epilepsy, Stol 1993: 119, 146). Thus, the transmission of negative – albeit invisible – properties, e.g. via physical intimacy or by association alone, was part of Mesopotamian thought. Regardless, one of the most cited passages concerning ancient contagion, and the rational means taken to avoid it, remains an Old Babylonian letter discovered at Mari from Zimri-Lim to his queen Šibtu regarding a woman named Nanna[4] who had taken ill, and the text states:

> "Now give strict orders, and (make sure) no one drinks of the cup, from which she drinks, no one sits on the chair, on which she sits, and that no one sleeps on the bed, upon which she sleeps. She should not gather (these) many women about herself! That wound (i.e., the epidemic) is *catching*."[5]

People in ancient Mesopotamia clearly had concrete ideas relating to contamination, though these were located somewhere at the intersection of magic, medicine, and religion. In the words of James Scott (2017: 106): "it was not until the late nineteenth-century discoveries of the founders of microbiology, Robert Koch and Louis Pasteur, that it became clear what a heavy price in chronic and lethal infections Homo sapiens was paying for the absence of clean water, sanitation, and sewage removal".[6]

The cuneiform sources available for researchers of epidemic history is rich, particularly because of the wide range of terms available for outlining ancient conceptualizations of such widespread sicknesses. Particularly two groups of sources are available to modern researchers, namely: (1) socio-political and historical documents; and (2) rituals, omen compendia, and mythological texts. In these texts, the terms for epidemics, in Akkadian or Sumerograms,[7] include the generic *mūtānu* (ÚŠ.MEŠ), a plural form of the word for "death", as well as more specialized terms from various periods, including the seasonal affliction *di'u/diḫu*,[8] DN *šumqutu* "DN strike down (with pestilence)", *kakki Erra* "the weapon of Erra", *lipit Erra*/DN "the touch of Erra/DN", *masla'tu*, *miqittu* (with several meanings in addition to epidemic), *qāt(i) Nergal* "the hand of Nergal", *simmu* any visible "wound", *šibṭu* "plague, epidemic", *šuruppû* "chills, shivers", *tīb(i) lemutti* "attack of plague" (and other meanings), and *ukulti* DN "the devouring by DN", derived from the verb *akālu* "to eat".[9] Despite this range of expressions, many terms remain understudied, and only a limited number of assyriological studies have collected the various sources to examine epidemic diseases and discussed responses to such times of crises.[10] In-

4 For the reading Nanna over Nanname, see the edition on Archibab no. 8685.

5 ARM 10 no. 129 rev. 10–u.e. 20, translation after Arbøll 2024: 18; for other recent translations with references to past literature, see the contributions by Attia and Heeßel in this volume.

6 The reasoning is probably right, though this is a truth with modifications. Many theories throughout history have attempted to shape human thought on how, when, and under which conditions diseases are able to spread, and some clearly had their roots in sensorial experiences connected to the eyes and nose regarding filth and decay. In the 18th century CE, for example, zymotic disease was introduced in between the older theory of miasma – connecting certain diseases to bad air – and the emergence of modern germ theory (McEnroe 2020: 1475). Zymotic diseases were contagious afflictions believed to develop within the body following an infection due to a process analogous to fermentation.

7 There appears to be few Sumerian terms, such as nam-úš, occasionally used to describe epidemics (see ePSD2: namuš [Death]).

8 Rites to keep this and similar epidemic afflictions from the door were performed in the winter months IX–XI in at least one instance in the Neo-Assyrian period to protect the court (see SAA 10 no. 296 obv. 11–rev. 1).

9 A number of terms that may refer to epidemic diseases include: *asakku*(?), *bibbu*(?), *dibiru*(?), *miširtu*(?), *namtaru*(?), and *šibbu*/*šībtu*(?).

10 E.g. Adamson 1982; Martinez 1990; von Weiher 2000; Heeßel 2009–10; Arbøll 2024; Couto-Ferreira 2024. Most articles present case studies, see Vanstiphout 1974; Vanstiphout 1980 Snell 1982; Neufeld 1986; Biggs 1991; Avalos 1995: 116–120; Çeçen 1995; Durand 1997; Klengel 1999; Farber 2004; Klinger 2012; Maul 2013; Singer 2017. For epidemics in Mari, see also Durand 1988: 544–549; LAPO 17: 471; LAPO 18: 187, 343–347; Charpin and Ziegler 2003: 111; Charpin 2015: 4. See Rashidi 2011 and Arbøll 2021 for general perspectives on zoonotic disease. See relevant Hittite rituals in Bawanypeck 2005; Cohen 2002: 55–56.

stead, researchers have invested considerable time in examining particularly the Late Bronze Age evidence from Mesopotamia, the Levant, Egypt, and Hittite Anatolia suggested to represent a single epidemic disease outbreak over the ancient Middle East.[11] Therefore, the topic of epidemics in ancient Mesopotamia has never been treated systematically beyond individual studies of select aspects, though a volume with individual articles focusing on Mesopotamia, edited by Jamieson et al. (2024) and entitled *Plague in Antiquity*, has recently been published. The present volume, however, represents the first monograph devoted solely to the study of Mesopotamian epidemics.

Many potentially rewarding avenues of research remain unexplored to examine ancient Near Eastern epidemic diseases, discussing ancient responses to times of crises, and examining epidemics on a general level, and a number of primary sources still require proper editions and discussions, specific terms must be analyzed, and various ideas regarding widespread disease should be reconsidered. For example, which tools did ancient specialists and everyday people have at their disposal for controlling such fearsome phenomena? And did they innovate these over the centuries? It is noticeable that very little narrative concerning plagues exist. Even the famous Poem of Erra and Išum (PEI) makes very few references to such events, though researchers tend to identify an apotropaic effect towards epidemics in the epic (see Arbøll in this volume). Likely, war was more manageable to describe, which also appears to be the case in PEI. Contrary to illness befallen an individual other than the king, disasters such as epidemics affected society at large. Still, it remains unclear if such events reflected poorly on rulers. In the context of epidemics, most rituals concern the household and beyond, and when they occasionally mention individuals, it appears to be the ruler. Many questions remain, for example it is not always clear if a precise aetiology always mattered,[12] how people reconciled the seemingly random disease patterns with the question "why me?",[13] if epidemics were generally considered cyclical and part of life,[14] and whether people imagined a remedy existed.[15]

This edited volume came about as a response to contemporary questions generated by the COVID-19 pandemic, and it represents the proceedings of a conference entitled *Infecting the Ancient Mesopotamian Cosmos*, which was held at the University of Oxford, Wolfson College, on the 29th to the 30th of April 2022. The intention of the gathering was to scrutinise the ancient terminology related to infection and illness, study the deities involved, examine concrete episodes of widespread disease and the impact of these, analyse changing perceptions of epidemics, study the ancient conceptualisation of contagion, assess inauspicious omens in relation to widespread sickness, the conceptualization of demons in relation to the death of animals, discuss ancient terms for epidemics, and consider how these were conceptualized in a cosmic setting. The speakers included Robert Arnott, Annie Attia, Barbara Böck, Eckart Frahm, Nils Heeßel, Adam Howe, Marta Iommelli, Ulla Koch, JoAnn Scurlock, as well as the editor of this volume.[16]

The proceedings in this volume are grouped according to three themes: (1) how the transmission of disease was understood in ancient Mesopotamia; (2) experiences of epidemic outbreaks and societal changes; and (3) ancient conceptualizations and understandings of epidemic outbreaks. In the first article in the initial section, Adam Howe explores demons as a conceptual tool for explaining and addressing contagious illnesses in relation to human waste. Marta Iommelli discusses the *samāna*- and *asakku*-demon as potential expressions for zoonotic disease concepts. Moving into the second section, Annie Attia examines primarily epistolary evidence, on the basis of which she outlines the visible effects of epidemics. Focusing on the Neo-Assyrian period, Eckart Frahm analyses the role of epidemic and pandemic outbreaks in relation to climate change and political crisis, and investigates how this explosive mix, somewhat counterintuitively, contributed to the Neo-Assyrian empire's consolidation in the 8th century BCE. Finally, in the third section Nils Heeßel examines the Babylonian astronomical diaries from the 1st millennium BCE to outline their role in comprehending and potentially predict ancient plagues. JoAnn Scurlock explores the gods Marduk and Nergal, and their roles

11 E.g. Singer 2017; Singer 2002: 56, 58; Klengel 1999; note the overly specific interpretation in Trevisanato 2007.

12 E.g. the Old Babylonian letter CT 29 pl. 1b = BM 28447, edited in AbB 2: 82–83 no. 118 and Pientka-Hinz 2006: 32–33, is concerned with correctly identifying the divine sender of an epidemic.

13 Which is what the Hittite plague prayers were intended to address in relation to the kingdom's ruler, see Singer 2002: 56, 58.

14 E.g. the epic narrative Atram-ḫasīs appears to argue for the existence of at least one such, intended to reduce humanity's numbers.

15 E.g. PEI appears to have served an apotropaic purpose to keep such afflictions away, and it may therefore be considered a remedy of sorts.

16 Though the speakers presented on a wide span of available sources and topics which can be studied as Mesopotamian epidemics, the proceedings here focus mainly on Assyria and Babylonia. Thus, they largely do not engage with Hittite sources, which might otherwise be able to provide additional insights into the question of "why me?" and similar aspects of ancient epidemics. It has not been possible to include these perspectives in this volume.

in ancient plague beliefs. Finally, Troels Arbøll provides the first study of the frequently used term *šibṭu* and its ancient conceptualization in relation to epidemic outbreaks.

It is the hope of the individual authors and this volume's editor that these contributions will facilitate further studies in the growing and contemporary field of Mesopotamian epidemics.

Bibliography

Adamson 1982 = P. B. Adamson, 'Human Diseases and Deaths in the Ancient Near East', *Die Welt des Orients* 13, 5–14

Avalos 1995 = H. Avalos, *Illness and Health Care in the Ancient Near East*, Harvard Semitic Monographs 54 (Atlanta: Scholars Press)

Arbøll 2024 = T. P. Arbøll, 'Revisiting Epidemics in Cuneiform Sources: Ancient Attestations, Approaches, and Innovations', in: *Plague in Antiquity*, ed. A. Jamieson, C. Tully, and L. Hitchcock, Ancient Near Eastern Studies Supplement Series (Leuven, Paris, and Walpole: Peeters), 13–33

Arbøll 2021 = T. P. Arbøll, 'Were People in Ancient Mesopotamia Aware of Zoonoses?', in: *Eskiçağda Salgın ve Hastalıklar*, ed. Ö. S. Gavaz and G. M. Şahin (Istanbul: Yayına Hazıirlayanlar), 23–50

Bawanypeck 2005 = D. Bawanypeck, *Die Rituale der Auguren*, Texte der Hethiter 25 (Heidelberg: Universitätsverlag Winter)

Biggs 1991 = R. D. Biggs, 'Ergotism and Other Mycotoxicoses in Ancient Mesopotamia?', *Aula Orientalis* 9, 15–21

Çeçen 1995 = S. Çeçen, '*mūtānu* in den Kültepe-Texten', *Archivum Anatolicum* 1, 43–72

Charpin 2015 = D. Charpin, 'La défaite, conséquence de la colère divine. La théologie de l'histoire à Alep d'après les archives royales de Mari', in: *Colères et repentirs divins*, ed. J.-M. Durand, L. Marti, and T. Römer, Orbis Biblicus et Orientalis 278 (Fribourg and Göttingen: Academic Press and Vandenhoeck & Ruprecht), 1–12

Charpin and Ziegler 2003 = D. Charpin and N. Ziegler, *Florilegium marianum V*, Mémoires de N.A.B.U. 6 (Antony: SEPOA)

Cohen 2002 = Y. Cohen, *Taboos and Prohibitions in Hittite Society* (Heidelberg: Universitätsvergal C. Winter)

Couto-Ferreira 2024 = E. Couto-Ferreira, 'Plagues and Epidemics in Ancient Mesopotamia: An Overview', in: Plague in Antiquity, ed. A. Jamieson, C. Tully, and L. Hitchcock, Ancient Near Eastern Studies Supplement Series (Leuven, Paris, and Walpole: Peeters), 49–62

Duggan et al. 2016 = A. T. Duggan, M. F. Perdomo, D. Piombino-Mascali, S. Marciniak, D. Poinar, M. V. Emery, J. P. Buchmann, S. Duchêne, R. Jankauskas, M. Humphreys, G. B. Golding, J. Southon, A. Devault, J.-M. Rouillard, J. W. Sahl, O. Dutoour, K. Hedman, A. Sajantila, G. L. Smith, E. C. Holmes, and H. N. Poinar, '17th Century Variola Virus Reveals the Recent History of Smallpox', *Current Biology* 26, 3407–3412

Durand 1988 = J.-M. Durand, *Archives Épistolaires de Mari 1/1*, Archives royales de Mari 26/1 (Paris: Librairie orientaliste Paul Geuthner)

Durand 1997 = J.-M. Durand, 'Les épidémies et les maladies', in: *Les documents épistolaires du palais de Mari*, ed. J.-M. Durand (Paris: Les Éditions du Cerf), 307–309

Ermidoro 2020 = S. Ermidoro, 'Animals in the Ancient Mesopotamian Diet. Prohibitions and Regulations Related to Meat in the First Millennium BCE', in: *Food Taboos and Biblical Prohibitions*, ed. P. Altmann, A. Angelini, and A. Spiciarich, Archaeology and Bible 2 (Tübingen: Mohr Siebeck), 25–42

Farber 2004 = W. Farber, 'How to Marry a Disease: Epidemics, Contagion, and a Magic Ritual Against the "Hand of the Ghost"', in: *Magic and Rationality in Ancient Near Eastern and Graeco-Roman Medicine*, ed. H. F. J. Horstmanshoff and M. Stol (Leiden and Boston: Brill), 117–132

Feder 2016 = Y. Feder, 'Defilement, Disgust, and Disease: The Experiential Basis of Hittite and Akkadian Terms for Impurity', *Journal of the American Oriental Society* 136/1, 99–116

Ferrari et al. 2020 = G. Ferrari, J. Neukamm, H. T. Baalsrud, A. M. Breidenstein, M. Ravinet, C. Phillips, F. Rühli, A. Bouwman, and V. J. Schuenemann, 'Variola virus genome sequenced from an eighteenth-century museum specimen supports the recent origin of smallpox', *Philosophical Transactions of the Royal Society B* 375, no. 20190572

Hardin 1993 = G. Hardin, *Living Within Limits: Ecology, Economics, and Population Taboos* (Oxford and New York: Oxford University Press)

Heeßel 2009–10 = N. P. Heeßel, 'Seuche', in: *Reallexikon der Assyriologie und Vorderasiatischen Archäologie. Band 12. Samuha–Sililitu*, ed. M. P. Streck (Berlin: De Gruyter), 405–406

Herring and Swedlund 2010 = D. A. Herring and A. C. Swedlund, *Plagues and Epidemics. Infected Spaces Past and Present* (London and New York: Routledge)

Jamieson et al. 2024 = A. Jamieson, C. Tully, and L. Hitchcock (eds.), *Plague in Antiquity*, Ancient Near Eastern Studies Supplement Series (Leuven, Paris, and Walpole: Peeters)

Jensen et al. 2019 = T. Z. T. Jensen, J. Niemann, K. H. Iversen, A. K. Fotakis, S. Gopalakrishnan, Å. J. Vågene, M. W. Pedersen, M.-H. S. Sinding, M. R. Ellegaard, M. E. Allentoft, L. T. Lanigan, A. J. Taurozzi, S. H. Nielsen, M. W. Dee, M. N. Mortensen, M. C. Christensen, S. A. Sørensen, M. J. Collins, M. T. P. Gilbert, M. Sikora, S. Rasmussen, and H. Schroeder, 'A 5700 year-old human genome and oral microbiome from chewed birch pitch', *Nature Communications* 10, Article number: 5520

Keck et al. 2019 = F. Keck, A. H. Kelly, and C. Lynteris, 'Introduction: the anthropology of epidemics', in: *The Anthropology of Epidemics*, ed. A. H. Kelly, F. Keck, and C. Lynteris, Routledge Studies in Health and Medical Anthropology (London and New York: Routledge), 1–24

Klengel 1999 = H. Klengel, 'Epidemien im spätbronzezeitlichen Syrien-Plästina', in: *Michael: Historical, Epigraphical and Biblical Studies in Honor of Prof. Michael Heltzer*, ed. Y. Avishur and R. Deutsch (Tel Aviv: Archaeological Center Publications), 187–193

Klinger 2012 = J. Klinger, 'Krankheit und Krieg im Spannungsfeld zwischen mythischer und realer Katastrophe', in: *Disaster and Relief Management*, ed. A. Berlejung, Forshungen zum Alten Testament 81 (Tübingen: Mohr Siebeck), 471–500

Martin and Martin-Granel 2006 = P. M. V. Martin and E. Martin-Granel, '2,500-year Evolution of the Term Epidemic', *Emerging Infectious Diseases* 12/6, 976–980

Martinez 1990 = R. M. Martinez, 'Epidemic Disease, Ecology, and Culture in the Ancient Near East', in: *The Bible in Light of Cuneiform Literature. Scripture in Context III*, ed. W. H. Hallo, B. W. Jones, and G. L. Mattingly, Ancient Near Eastern Texts and Studies 8 (Lewiston, Queenston, and Lampeter: Edwin Mellen Press), 413–457

Maul 2013 = S. M. Maul, 'Ein altorientalischer Pferdesegen – Seuchenprophylaxe in der assyrischen Armee', *Zeitschrift für Assyriologie* 103/1, 16–37

McEnroe 2020 = N. McEnroe, 'The art of medicine. Celebrating Florence Nightingale's bicentenary', *The Lancet* 395, 1475–1478

Mühlemann et al. 2020 = B. Mühlemann, L. Vinner, A. Margaryan, H. Wilhelmson, C. F. Castro, M. E. Allentoft, P. B. Damgaard, A. J. Hansen, S. H. Nielsen, L. M. Strand, J. Bill, A. Buzhilova, T. Pushkina, C. Falys, V. Khartanovich, V. Moiseyev, M. L. S. Jørkov, P. Ø. Sørensen, Y. Magnusson, I. Gustin, H. Schroeder, G. Sutter, G. L. Smith, C. Drosten, R. A. M. Fouchier, D. J. Smith, E. Willerslev, T. C. Jones, and M. Sikora, 'Diverse virola virus (smallpox) strains were widespread in northern Europe in the Viking Age', *Science* 369, DOI: 10.1126/science.aaw8977

Nemeroff and Rozin 2000 = C. Nemeroff and P. Rozin, 'The Makings of the Magical Mind", in: *Imagining the Impossible*, ed. K. S. Rosengren, C. N. Johnson, and L. Harris (Cambridge: Cambridge University Press), 1–34

Neufeld 1986 = E. Neufeld, 'The Earliest Document of a Case of Contagious Disease in Mesopotamia (Mari Tablet *ARM* X, 129)', *Journal of the Ancient Near Eastern Society* 18, 53–66

Nielsen et al. 2021 = S. H. Nielsen, L. van Dorp, C. J. Houldcroft, A. G. Pedersen, M. E. Allentoft, L. Vinner, A. Margaryan, E. Pavlova, V. Chasnyk, P. Nikolskiy, V. Pitulko, V. N. Pimenoff, F. Balloux, and M. Sikora, '31,600-year-old human virus genomes support a Pleistocene origin for common childhood infections', *bioRxiv*, https://doi.org/10.1101/2021.06.28.450199

Pientka-Hinz 2006 = R. Pientka-Hinz, 'Altbabylonische Briefe', in: *Texte aus der Umwelt des Alten Testaments. Neue Folge. Band 3. Briefe* (Gütersloh: Gütersloher Verlagshaus), 21–37

Rashidi 2011 = J. S. Rashidi, *Paleoepidemiology of Mesopotamia and the Ancient Near East: The Impact of Zoonotic Diseases and Population Demographics on Infectious Disease Patterns* [PhD Dissertation] (Los Angeles)

Rasmussen et al. 2015 = S. Rasmussen, M. E. Allentoft, K. Nielsen, L. Orlando, M. Sikora, K.-G. Sjögren, A. G. Pedersen, M. Schubert, A. van Dam, C. M. O. Kapel, H. B. Nielsen, S. Brunak, P. Avetisyan, A. Epimakhov, M. V. Khalyapin, A. Gnuni, A. Kriiska, I. Lesak, M. Metspalu, V. Moiseyev, A. Gromov, D. Pokutta, L. Saag, L. Varul, L. Yepiskoposyan, T. Sicheritz-Pontén, R. A. Foley, M. M. Lahr, R. Nielsen, K. Kristiansen, and E. Willerslev, 'Early Divergent Strains of *Yersinia pestis* in Eurasia 5,000 Years Ago', *Cell* 163/3, 571–582

Rosenberg 1992 = C. E. Rosenberg, Explaining Epidemics and Other Studies in the History of Medicine (Cambridge: Cambridge University Press)

Salin 2015 = S. Salin, 'When Disease "Touches", "Hits", or "Seizes" in Assyro-Babylonian Medicine', *Kaskal* 12, 319–336

Scheidel 2017 = W. Scheidel, *The Great Leveler. Violence and the History of Inequality from the Stone Age to the Twenty-First Century* (Princeton and Oxford: Princeton University Press)

Scott 2017 = J. C. Scott, *Against the Grain. A Deep History of the Earliest States* (New Haven and London: Yale University Press)

Singer 2017 = G. G. Singer, 'Beyond Amarna: The "Hand of Nergal" and the Plague in the Levant', *Ugarit Forschungen* 48, 223–247

Singer 2002 = I. Singer, *Hittite Prayers*, Writings from the Ancient World 11 (Atlanta: Society of Biblical Literature)

Snell 1982 = D. Snell, 'Plagues and Peoples in Mesopotamia', *Journal of the Ancient Near Eastern Society* 14, 89–96

Snowden 2020 = F. Snowden, *Epidemics and Society. From the Black Death to the Present* [Paperback Edition] (New Haven and London: Yale University Press)

Spernovasilis et al. 2021 = N. Spernovasilis, I. Markaki, M. Papadakis, C. Tsioutis, and L. Markaki, 'Epidemics and pandemics: Is human overpopulation the elephant in the room?', *Ethics, Medicine and Public Health* 19, DOI: 10.1016/j.jemep.2021.100728

Stol 1993 = M. Stol, *Epilepsy in Babylonia*, Cuneiform Monographs 2 (Groningen: Styx Publications)

Sørensen 2007 = J. Sørensen, A Cognitive Theory of Magic (Lanham, New York, Toronto, and Plymouth: Altamira Press)

van der Toorn 1985 = K. van der Toorn, *Sin and Sanction in Israel and Mesopotamia*, Studia Semitica Neerlandica 22 (Assen and Maastricht: Van Gorcum)

Trevisanato 2007 = S. I. Trevisanato, 'The "Hittite plague', an epidemic of tularemia and the first record of biological warfare', *Medical Hypotheses* 69, 1371–1374

United Nations [Anonymous author] 2022: "Biodiversity – our strongest natural defence against climate change", <https://www.un.org/en/climate change/science/climate-issues/biodiversity> (accessed 04/06/2024)

Vanstiphout 1974 = H. L. J. Vanstiphout, 'Was een pestepidemie de oorzaak van de ondergang von het Nieuwsumerische rijk?', *Phoenix* 20, 351–370

Vanstiphout 1980 = H. L. J. Vanstiphout, 'The "Great Mortality" in the Sumerian City Lamentations', in: *Death in Mesopotamia. XXVIe Recontre assyriologique internationale*, ed. B. Alster, Mesopotamia 8 (Copenhagen: Akademisk Forlag), 83–89

von Weiher 2000 = E. von Weiher, 'Seuchen und Pest im Alten Orient', in: *Heilkunde und Hochkultur I: Geburt, Seuche und Traumdeutung in den antiken Zivilisationen des Mittelmeerraumes*, ed. A. Karenberg and C. Leitz (Münster, Hamburg, and London: LIT Verlag), 47–54

Yeomans et al. 2024 = L. Yeomans, M. C. Codlin, C. Mazzucato, F. D. Bello, and B. Demarchi, 'Waterfowl eggshell refines palaeoenvironmental reconstruction and supports multi-species niche construction at the Pleistocene-Holocene transition in the Levant', *Journal of Archaeological Method and Theory*, https://doi.org/10.1007/s10816-024-09641-0

1 The transmission of infectious diseases

Adam Howe

Dirty Demons: Sewage, Rubbish, and Pollution as Sources of Contagion in Udug-ḫul

In incantations of the Mesopotamian exorcistic corpus, the imagery of demons is frequently employed as a means of conceptualizing otherwise invisible or incomprehensible dangers posed by the world around us. In this way, abstract fears could be translated into a more concrete and "ritually controllable form" that could be targeted by the exorcist's rituals.[1] As well as embodying numerous diseases and other health conditions, demons could be invoked as manifestations or causes of various environmental dangers. In the extensive anti-demon ritual Udug-ḫul,[2] this includes life-threatening weather conditions,[3] invisible dangers of the marshland like malaria,[4] undesirable or ill-omened creatures,[5] and perhaps even the threat of brush fires, venomous spiders, and rotting fruit.[6] Many of these dangers come from the natural world and are especially associated with the steppe: the environment beyond and between urban and cultivated areas was largely uncontrolled by humans and therefore presented a number of dangers, both human and otherwise. Due to these dangers and its liminal position within the human-centered world, the steppe was particularly identified as the dwelling place of demons, who are often portrayed roaming the steppe preying on unfortunate victims.[7] Rituals against demons make clear, however, that the threat of demons was not restricted to the steppe but that they could also pursue humans into the urban environment and even into their homes, taking advantage of vulnerable openings such as doors, windows, bathroom drains, and gaps or cracks in the building fabric.[8] Demons could therefore pose a threat even in supposedly safe urban and domestic environments, but fortunately there were plenty of ritual measures available to the Mesopotamian exorcist to contend with this threat.

This paper examines how the writings of these exorcists employed the imagery of demons to represent not only the dangers posed by the untamed natural world but also the relatively novel dangers of living in a densely populated urban environment. It focuses in particular on the role of demons as a conceptual tool for addressing potential contagions and infectious illness arising from the accumulation of human waste. It will consider how this waste, in the form of sewage and household refuse, both of which were potentially dangerous to human health, could have been dealt with in a Mesopotamian context. This includes, of course, physical interventions into the built environment such as

1 This terminology is adapted from Schwemer (2007: 147) who frames Mesopotamian witchcraft beliefs as a way of allowing "die eigenen Ängste, die Konflikte mit den Mitmenschen und die damit einhergehenden Aggressionen in einer rituell kontrollierten Form zu artikulieren".
2 Henceforth abbreviated to UH, and cited after the edition of Geller (2016), unless otherwise stated.
3 E.g. UH IV 36–39: "They are great storms, *Utukku*-demons who roam about, who destroy the land, they do not spare the bricks of the treasury, they make the mountain roar like a porous vessel"; UH XVI 14–16: "They are the dust storms that circle about furiously in the sky, they are the dense clouds that cause gloominess in the sky, they are the blast of rising wind that causes darkness on a bright day". Also prominent in Udug-ḫul are the "Day-Demons" (u_4 // *ūmu*), whose malevolent forms are usually associated with the storm god and who descend from heaven as storms (Wiggermann 1992: 171).
4 UH XIII–XV 11–12: "They are the terror in the marsh, they are the Asakku-demon in the reedbed". Due to its association with illnesses characterized by extremes of temperature, the Asakku-demon has been identified as a personification of malaria (Bácskay 2017: 50).
5 E.g. UH V 9: "They are the owl that cries out in the city"; UH VI 174′–176′: "They constantly slither about by themselves like a snake, they sniff at the sewage outlet like a mongoose, they roam about like stray dogs"; UH VIII 18–19, 23: "Whether you are the *Alû*-demon who constantly flies around at night in crevices like a bat, or you are the *Alû*-demon who constantly flies about in the darkness like a night-bird, . . ., or you are the *Alû*-demon who prowls silently at night like an urban fox".
6 UH XIII–XV 13–15: "They are the igniting of embers in the forest (Sum. they set a torch to the forest (?)), they are the evil (spider's?) web in the mouth of a jar, they are the forgotten (Sum. *plundered*) fruit in the orchards". These last two lines, if interpreted correctly, demonstrate how dangers from the natural environment, like demons, can encroach upon human society.
7 In this way, demons could also be compared to human threats in the steppes, such as bandits (e.g. UH V 146: "*Rābisu*-demon (lit. 'lurker') of the road and highway") and murderers (e.g. UH III 31: "The evil *Utukku*-demon who murders a healthy man in the steppe"). See further Fincke 2013.
8 UH IX lines 89′–110′, and the similar passages ASKT 11 lines 166–202 and Saĝ-ba I lines 41–120, enumerate various parts of the house that were vulnerable to demons, with the ASKT 11 passage repeating a refrain addressed to the demon: "Do not enter to him!" (nam-mu-un-du-ku_4-ku_4-de_3 // *lā terrubšu*).

Adam Howe, Philipps-Universität Marburg

 | https://doi.org/10.1515/9783112238622-002

drainage or rubbish dumps, but also the possibility of conceptualizing the dangers in terms of demons, which provided a more suitable target for ritual protective measures and a means of explaining the threat. The paper concludes with a close reading of a difficult passage involving sewage and watercourses from Udug-ḫul 11, also known as Marduk's Address to the Demons, offering a possible interpretation in light of the preceding discussion.

1 Waste Management in Ancient Mesopotamia

Urbanization was characteristic of life in Mesopotamia since before the dawn of writing but, at least until the advent of modern public healthcare and sanitation, life in cities posed an unprecedented threat to the health of their inhabitants, leading to high levels of mortality and a situation described as the "paradox of urbanism".[9] Not only did the densification of human populations increase the impact of infectious illness,[10] but various Mesopotamian sources also recognize the potential contagiousness of the accumulation of human effluence.[11] Measures taken against this included ritualized cleaning, making sweeping the house into a form of apotropaic ritual to keep potential contagions away,[12] or burying apotropaic figurines at the entrance to the bathroom to keep demons at bay.[13] Very occasionally, physical interventions were also made into the built environment, namely sewage systems and centralized rubbish disposal, with the intention of not only removing waste but also keeping it separate from parts of houses and the wider city that were usually frequented by people.

While many inhabitants of Mesopotamia may simply have gone to the toilet outside,[14] there are textual references to a part of the house called the *bīt musâti*, literally 'house of (dirty) wash-water', which is usually identified as the lavatory or bathroom, even if not much detail is given in the ancient textual sources regarding its form or function.[15] In the archaeological record, rooms with a similar function are usually identified on the basis of being connected to some sort of drainage system for disposing of the contaminated water produced there.[16] While apparently never particularly widespread,[17] there is archaeological evidence from Mesopotamia for two types of drainage or waste disposal system connected to houses: the deep-pit toilet and the sloped-drain toilet. Deep pit toilets are attested from the 4th millennium BCE onwards and consist of interlocking ceramic rings tapering to a smaller hole at the top, with the spaces in between filled with sherds.[18] These would have easily filled up over the use-life of building, so they either had to have some way of being emptied or were possibly only used for liquid waste, which would have seeped into the surrounding soil.[19]

Sloped-drain toilets, on the other hand, were primarily a feature of larger elite dwellings, including first-millennium BCE Assyrian palaces,[20] and would presumably have been familiar to the exorcists working with the anti-demon rituals discussed below (see Figure 1). This type of toilet simply flushed waste out into the street, probably with rainwater, which would have helped to keep the pipes from becoming blocked but also created a pool of contaminated water in the street, thereby increasing the risk of disease transmission. The outlet to the street is probably the feature

9 Algaze 2018.

10 Cf. Tenney 2017: 735.

11 Cf. Scurlock and Andersen 2005: 19. For example, a bilingual hemerology suggests entering a toilet could result in abdominal illness (Cavigneaux and Al-Rawi 1993: 102, 16–17), while a medical text cites treading in dirty wash-water as a cause of a foot condition (Eypper 2016: 12, i 18).

12 Scurlock and Andersen 2005: 15; Maul 1994: 500, 28–30.

13 George 2015: 90.

14 McMahon 2015: 21. The toilet demon Šulak is also said to be a threat in date-groves and deserted places, where people may well have gone to the toilet for want of a dedicated space (George 2015: 88).

15 George 2015: 86; McMahon 2015: 20–21.

16 E.g. Reuther 1929: 95, 111–112. For an overview of the archaeology of plumbing and drains in the ancient Near East, see Hemker 1993: 168–173, and for Mesopotamian toilets in particular, see Krafeld-Daugherty 1994: 95–112 and McMahon 2015: 22–31.

17 At most sites, density of toilet or drainage installations is fairly low (McMahon 2015: 25–27).

18 McMahon 2015: 22–23.

19 McMahon 2015: 25. Street channels found in Neo-Babylonian Babylon, for example, could have been used to empty deep-pit toilets from neighboring houses (Reuther 1926: 76).

20 McMahon 2015: 30.

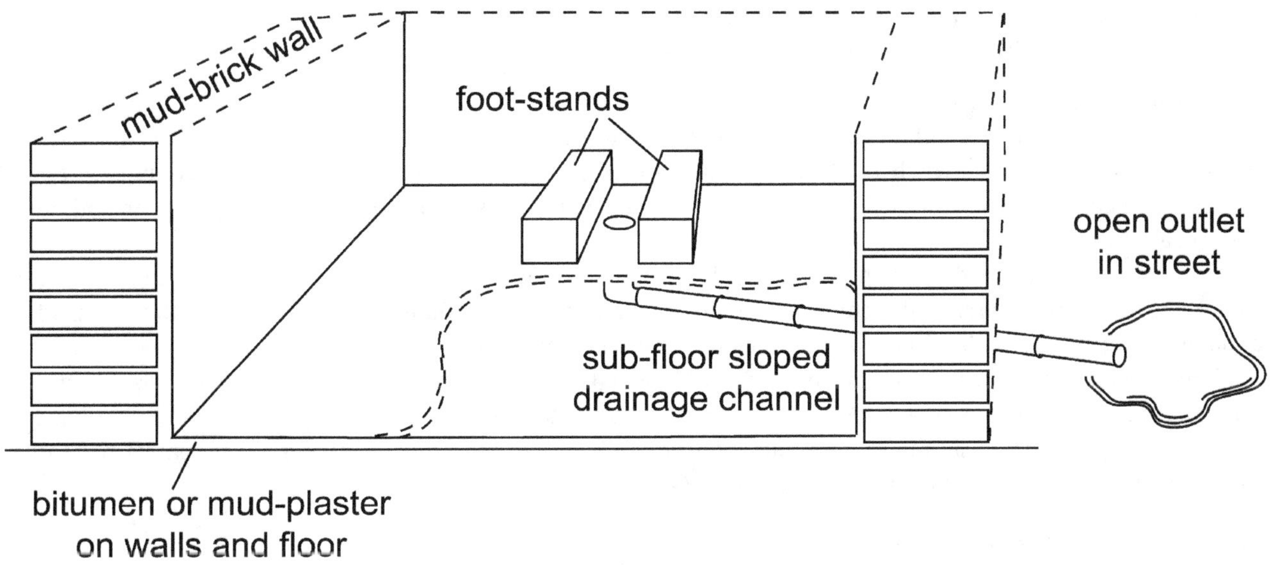

Figure 1: Diagram of a typical sloped-drain toilet as attested from 3rd millennium BCE Mesopotamia (McMahon 2015: 29, fig. 3.3).

denoted by Akkadian *asurrû*, which Andrew George has demonstrated to refer to a 'sewage outlet'.[21] The *asurrû* was a sort of hollow pipe, since snakes and mongooses could get inside, which opened out onto the street, since an incantation against stomach ache describes pigs sniffing around it.[22] It must have been connected to an interior part of the house if it was also a way by which demons could get in, and thus it is this sort of drainage system that is relevant to the discussion here. Nevertheless, dedicated toilets and drainage systems were likely extremely rare, and other methods such as portable containers and defecating outside would leave no trace in the archaeological record.[23] Such methods raise the possibility of the secondary use of human waste as manure, but there is no evidence for its organized collection and this would not have removed the risks to public health.[24] Whether or not the waste issuing from drains was eventually removed from the streets, the associations between demons and toilets and drains in exorcistic texts demonstrate that human effluence was seen as dangerous, especially to the elite clients of the exorcists, even though they could probably afford to remove it from their homes in a relatively hygienic way.

Other household waste was ideally disposed of at a distance from the place of habitation, and there is evidence for the existence of communal rubbish dumps, although it is not possible to establish whether these were instituted by a centralized authority or simply arose organically out of necessity. The state of a city's rubbish dump is referenced in terrestrial omens as an indicator of the wellbeing of the city (e.g. *Šumma ālu* 1 35–37, 47–49):

35 *šumma*(diš) *ālu*(uru) *tub*$_2$-*qi*$_2$-*na-šu*$_2$ *iš-qu ālu*(uru) *šū*(bi) *innaddi*(šub)^{di}
36 *šumma*(diš) *ālu*(uru) MIN(= *tubqinnašu*) *išātu*(izi) *ālu*(uru) *šū*(bi) *mūtānu*(uš$_2$)^{meš} *ittanaddi*(šub)^{meš}-*šu*$_2$
37 *šumma*(diš) *ālu*(uru) MIN(= *tubqinnašu*) *elēnu*(an.ta)^{nu} *šaknat*(gar)^{at} *ālu*(uru) *šū*(bi) *inaddi*(šub)^{di}
35 If a city's rubbish dump has become high: that city will be abandoned.
36 If fire consumes a city's rubbish dump: plague will constantly befall that city.
37 If a city's rubbish dump is sited upstream: that city will be abandoned.
47 *šumma*(diš) *ālu*(uru) MIN(= *tubqinnašu*) *kīma*(gin$_7$) *ka-a-pi nāra*(id$_2$) *u*$_2$-*kal ālu*(uru) *šū*(bi) *lemnu*(ḫul) *iṣabbat*(dab)-*su*
48 *šumma*(diš) *ālu*(uru) MIN(= *tubqinnašu*) *šaplat ālu*(uru) *šū*(bi) *šubat*(ki.tus) *nēḫti*(ne.ḫa) *uššab*(dur$_2$)^{ab}
49 [*šumma*(diš)] *ālu*(uru) MIN(= *tubqinnašu*) *ra-aq ālu*(uru) *šū*(bi) ŠU.BI.AŠ.AM$_3$
47 If a city's rubbish dump holds back the river like an embankment: evil will seize that city.

21 George 1999: 551; 2015: 90–98. The Akkadian seems to be based on an otherwise unattested Sumerian form a-sur-ra, literally 'water discharger' (George 2015: 98).
22 George 2015: 93–96.
23 McMahon 2015: 32.
24 McMahon 2015: 33–34.

48 If a city's rubbish dump is low: that city will dwell in peace.
49 [If] a city's rubbish dump is empty: that city *ditto* (i.e. will dwell in peace).[25]

The logic behinds these omens is fairly self-evident, but they demonstrate a recognition of the potential danger that the disposal of waste could pose to public health. These rubbish dumps were considered places to be avoided, usually frequented by dogs, demons, and witches.[26] However, with a lack of organized refuse collection, these dumps were not necessarily located outside or at the edge of settlements as today, but most people probably dumped their household waste in nearby streets or alleys.[27]

Due in part to their danger to health and association with undesirable beings, these places for dumping waste were an important part of the exorcist's discourse, and in literary sources rubbish dumps are referred to with the Akkadian term *tub/pk/qinnu*.[28] The rubbish dump was an obvious place for disposing of contaminated or magically charged materials, although being public it was not entirely secure. A witch, for example, could use a rubbish dump as a source of materials for manipulating her victim.[29] Exorcists themselves could take advantage of this, placing representations of a patient's suffering on a rubbish dump in the hope that it would be carried off by an unsuspecting passer-by. This is described in the incantation known as *attī tubkinni* (79–7–8, 71 7′–12′):

7′ [EN$_2$ *at-ti*] *tub-kin-ni *ma{maḫ}*-ḫi-rat ka-la mim-ma šum-*[*šu*]
8′ [*ni-šu ta*]*-maḫ-ḫa-ri ma-mit ta-maḫ-ḫa-*[*ri*]
9′ [*tur-ta ta*]*-maḫ-ḫa-ri maš-al-ti ta-maḫ-ḫa-*[*ri*]
10′ [*li-i*'*-bu*] ⸢*ta*⸣*-ma-ḫa-ru um-ma ta-*⸢*maḫ*⸣-[*ḫa-ri*]
11′ [*muruṣ*(gig) *ta-ne*$_2$]-⸢*ḫu*?⸣ *ar*$_2$*-ni šer*$_3$*-ti gil*$_2$*-la-ti ḫi-ṭi-ti* [*tamaḫḫarī*(?)]
12′ [*e-ti-qu*$_2$*-ki lim-ḫu*]-⸢*ru*⸣*-in-ni ka-bi-su-ki li-tin-nu-u* [*itti*(ki)*-ia*]
7′ [Incantation: You] (are) the rubbish dump who receives everything,
8′ [you] receive [oath], you receive curse,
9′ [you] receive ['turning'], you receive 'questioning',
10′ you receive [*li'bu*-fever], you receive *ummu*-fever,
11′ [you receive(?) wailing illness], crime, offence, sin, error,
12′ [may whoever passes you] receive (all this) for me, may whoever treads on you change (places) [with me].[30]

The various evils, impurities, and illnesses afflicting the patient are formulaically listed as being received by or passed on to the rubbish dump.[31] The ritual then relies on the fact that someone passing the rubbish dump might themselves come into contact with the impure materials and carry them off again,[32] whether this was someone unsuspectingly dumping their own waste or a marginalized person eking out their existence from others' waste.[33] Rubbish dumps were thus not universally avoided, and their function in exorcistic rituals revolves around their being a place where contagion could be both disposed of and encountered. From a Mesopotamian perspective, however, this contagion was not

25 Text after Project Ālu Geneva composite edition, available through the electronic Babylonian Library <www.ebl.lmu.de/corpus/D/2/2/SB/1> (accessed 25/01/2023). Cf. Freedman 1998: 28–29.
26 Greenfield and Schafer 1983: 125–126.
27 McMahon 2015: 34.
28 This seems to be a deverbal noun derived from *tabāku* 'to pour out' on the *pursennu* pattern of pejorative diminutives (Greenfield and Schafer 1983: 125, cf. GAG § 56r). Note that the term is still frequently confused in the modern literature with *tubqu* 'corner' (cf. Biggs 1993).
29 *Maqlû* II 186: *ina tub-kin-na-ti u*$_2$*-laq-qi*$_2$*-tu ḫu-ṣa-be*$_2$*-e-a* "(The witch who) gathered my leavings (lit. splinters) from rubbish dumps". Given that *ḫuṣābu* literally just means 'something broken off', it may refer here to general household waste that has come into contact with the victim or to the sort of biological materials (e.g. fingernail clippings, armpit hair, urine) that the witch could use for magical manipulation.
30 Previously edited in Van der Toorn 1985: 138–139, with collations by the present author from the photograph on CDLI <cdli.ucla.edu/P451822> (accessed 26/04/2022). Restorations in the final line follow a similar passage in *Bīt rimki* (Læssøe 1955: 58–59, 92–94): *erṣetu*(ki)*tu lim-ḫur-an-ni lid-di-na melamma*(me.lam$_2$)*-ša*$_2$*-ma lum-ni lit-bal* / ⸢*ka*⸣*-bi-su erṣeta*(ki) *lim-ḫu-ru-nin-ni* / ⸢*e*⸣*-ti-qu erṣeta*(ki) *li-tin-nu-u itti*(ki)*-ia* "May the earth receive (the impurities) for me, may it give me its *melammu* and carry off my evil, may (anyone) who treads on (this piece of) earth receive (the impurities) for me, may (anyone) who passes (this piece of) earth change (places) with me".
31 The verb *maḫāru* can be used to describe the transfer of contagion or portended evil (cf. CAD M/1 59).
32 A similar practice is found in an anti-witchcraft ritual, in which a money-bag containing precious metals and stones is offered to Šamaš, but also abandoned in the hope that a passer-by will pick it up and carry off the witchcraft's evil (CMAwR 8.2 26–27, 38, 122; see Abusch and Schwemer 2011: 256 for this interpretation of the ritual).
33 That this practice was known in Mesopotamia is suggested by one of the curses in the Tell Fekheriye bilingual inscription (Abou-Assaf et al. 1982: 14, 36–37): . . . *eli*(ugu) *tub-ki-na-te la-qi-te* / *lil-qu-te* . . . "May they scavenge for scraps on the rubbish dumps".

understood to be caused by bacteria but by the fact that ritual and cultic pollution could be transmitted by contact with already afflicted people and objects[34]

In later periods, it seems that dedicated systems for managing sewage became even less common, with wastewater often simply flushed under the thresholds of houses into the street.[35] At the same time, the majority of households probably dumped other household waste within their houses or in nearby streets,[36] with the thresholds of buildings regularly being raised to keep all of this waste at least somewhat separated from the home environment.[37] In the streets, the waste would have been eaten by free-roaming animals like dogs and pigs, which would in turn have contributed to the build-up of waste in the street with their excrement.[38] The average Mesopotamian city-dweller would therefore have been confronted by dangerous, potentially contagious waste as soon as they stepped out of their front door. It is no surprise that evil forces like witches and demons were believed to roam the streets alongside animals and marginalized humans, using them to gain access from the outside world into people's private spaces.

2 Demons and household waste

The threat that sewage and other household waste posed to the health and wellbeing of individuals and the community as a whole was recognized in Mesopotamia, and certain concrete steps were taken to protect against it. With little understanding of germ theory, such measures would have had limited success, so the section of society whose viewpoint is represented in the exorcistic texts would also conceptualize these largely invisible and intangible dangers in terms of demons. This would have provided a more concrete target for counteractive rituals and perhaps also functioned as a way of encouraging the responsible disposal and treatment of household waste. Indeed, in various anti-demon incantations, demons are often associated with sewage, drains, rubbish dumps, and other sources of contamination. In Udug-ḫul, for example, demons are described being attracted to sewage outlets like mongooses (UH IV 175′):

> ^{d}nin-kilim-gin$_7$ ur$_2$ e$_2$-gar$_8$-ra-ke$_4$ ir-si-im in-na-AK-e-de$_3$
> *ki-ma šik-ke-e a-sur-ra-a uṣ-ṣa-nu šu-nu*
> They sniff at the sewage outlet (Sumerian: base of the wall)[39] like the mongoose.

As discussed above, the *asurrû* is presumably a feature of the sloped-drain type toilets, or a channel running beneath the threshold of houses, both of which drained waste directly into the street. The demons are thus imagined sniffing at the opening to the drain or the dirty water pooled around it, presumably using the distinctive smell of the drain to locate a vulnerable point of entry to a person's house.[40] This forms part of the portrayal of demons as beings opposed to the norms of human society, attracted to something that should be repulsive, but also represents how demons could take advantage of humans' biological vulnerabilities to attack them. In this way, demons served as a means of addressing fears about contagion and vulnerable situations like going to the toilet.

Fear of the vulnerability inherent in this biological imperative is exemplified by the demon known as Šulak. Šulak was associated especially with the *bīt musâti* and sometimes has the epithet *rābiṣ musâti* 'lurker of the (dirty) washwater'.[41] Šulak and the Hand of Šulak were held responsible for a variety of medical conditions, but especially stroke, which it was apparently believed could be caused by straining too hard on the toilet.[42] Another aspect of Šulak to recog-

---

34 Cf. Feder 2016: 110; 2022: 40–42.

35 As, for example, in Middle and Neo-Assyrian Assur (Preusser 1954: 63).

36 McMahon (2015: 38) notes that rubbish dumps attested in the archaeological record primarily contain elite objects and are probably to be associated with wealthier households which could afford to have their waste transported further away from where they lived.

37 Steinert 2014: 142.

38 E.g. Lambert 1960: 215 (KAR 174) rev. iii 13–14: "The pig is not holy [(. . .) smear]ing (its) backside, making the streets smell, polluting the houses". This function of pigs may have contributed to the avoidance of consuming pork in the ancient Near East, but the precise reasons for this are not clear and the practice was hardly universal (cf. Welton 2020: 87–91).

39 The Sumerian reflects a later semantic development of Akkadian *asurrû*, which can refer to the base of the wall more generally (George 2015: 99–102). With the references to sniffing mongooses, however, it must refer to the sewage outlet here.

40 Cf. George 2015: 94.

41 George 2015: 89; Stol 1993: 76.

42 George 2015: 88.

nize the health risks of using the bathroom is the folk etymology, attested in a commentary from Uruk, that interprets the demon's name as meaning 'dirty hands' (i.e. šu *lā* ku$_3$).[43] This suggests an awareness of the possibility of contagion from human effluence and poor hygiene, and how the actions of demons were projected onto these genuine threats to health, with the source of contagion effectively being equated with the demon. In this way, bathroom hygiene could in theory be managed with measures against the demon. For example, apotropaic figurines representing the *urmaḫlullû* lion-man are mentioned in ritual texts as guards against the leonine demon Šulak and such figurines have indeed been found buried near the entrances to bathrooms in Assyrian palaces.[44]

It is possible that Šulak and other demons associated with the toilet also reflect fears about the possibility of dangerous animals entering through the drains, a fear that circulates widely today even if it is usually nothing more than an urban legend.[45] It is common for demons to be described entering their victim's home through various vulnerable openings, including windows, the eaves of the roof, parts of the door, and of course the drains, as in this passage from the zi-pa$_3$ incantation ASKT 11 (179–180):

179 pu$_2$-ta nam(-mu-un-da-ku$_4$-ku$_4$-de$_3$)
[*ina*] ⸢*bur*⸣-*ti* MIN(= *lā terrubšu*)
180 pu$_2$ du$_{10}$-us$_2$-sa-ta nam(-mu-un-da-ku$_4$-ku$_4$-de$_3$)
[*ina*] *bur-tu$_4$ nar-ma-ki* MIN(= *lā terrubšu*)
179 Do not enter to him through the cistern!
180 Do not enter to him through the bathing-cistern![46]

These two types of well or cistern, with one perhaps for drinking water and the other for bathing, must have been dug into the foundations of the house. In a similar but expanded passage from the series Saĝ-ba, a demon is described 'coming up' from these cisterns and they are compared to a pitfall trap (I 95–102):

95 pu$_2$-ta mu-ni-ib$_2$-e$_{11}$-de$_3$
96 *ša$_2$ ul-tu bur-ti il-la-a*
97 ub$_4$ niĝ$_2$-ḫuš-a-ta ḫe$_2$-ni-ib$_2$-šub-bu-ne
98 *a-na šu-ut-ta-ti lid-du-šu$_2$*
99 ⸢pu$_2$⸣ du$_{10}$-us$_2$-sa-a-ta mu-un-gir$_5$-gir$_3$-e-de$_3$
100 *ša$_2$ ina bur-ti nar-ma-ki i-ḫal-lu-pu*
101 pu$_2$ nu-e$_{11}$-da-ta ḫe$_2$-ni-ib$_2$-šub-bu-ne
102 *ana bur-ti la-a-le-e lid-du-šu$_2$*
95 That which comes up from the cistern,
97 may they throw it into a pitfall!
99 That which slips in through the bathing-cistern,
101 may they throw it into a cistern from which there is no coming up![47]

It is no surprise that a dark hole where dangerous animals like snakes and mongooses, as well as scorpions,[48] might have been hiding should have been feared as a haunt of demons.[49] If some of these drains emptied out into the street, they also created a connection between the house and the outside world, offering demons a potential access point to attack their victim in the safety of their own home. Additionally, some of the fear must be connected to the inherent

43 George 2015: 89, citing SpTU I 47, 2–5.
44 Wiggermann 1992: 86; 98.
45 See e.g. <www.bbc.co.uk/news/magazine-36397505> (accessed 27/01/2023) for a discussion of which animals might or might not find their way into your toilet. Nevertheless, urban legends are perhaps an appropriate modern parallel to Mesopotamian demon beliefs, since they also act as something onto which fears about society and the world around us are projected and thereby processed.
46 Borger 1969: 10.
47 Schramm 2001: 24–25; 54–55.
48 Marten Stol (2020: 570) has identified the *alap asurrê*, literally 'ox of the sewage outlet', referenced in BAM 244 rev. 44 as a type of scorpion, possibly representing the demon Šulak.
49 Cf. McMahon 2015: 21.

vulnerability of the acts of going to the toilet or bathing, also reflected in the fact that ghosts could attack their victims in the bath,[50] or that Šulak could attack people going to the toilet anywhere.

The rubbish dump too was a liminal and dangerous place that was best avoided as far as possible, but it was also somewhere where witches and exorcists were active for their own reasons. Unsurprisingly, the rubbish dump, along with the sewage outlet, is also identified in Udug-ḫul as a place where demons might be lurking (UH XI 17′–21′):

17′ *lu-u ša*$_2$ *bītāti*(e$_2$)^{meš} *te-te-ne*$_2$*-er-ru-ba*
18′ *lu-u*$_2$ *ša*$_2$ *as-kup-pa-a-ti teš-te-ni-ʾi-ra*
19′ [*lu-u ša*$_2$] ⸢*ūrī*(ur$_3$)⸣[^{meš}] ⸢*tat*⸣*-ta-nab-lak-ka-tu*
20′ *lu-u ša*$_2$ *ina a-sur-re-e ta-at-ta-na-al-la-ka*
21′ *lu-u ša*$_2$ *ina tub-qi-na-a-ti ta-at-ta-na-aš*$_2$*-ša*$_2$*-ba*
17′ Whether (you are ones) who constantly enter houses,
18′ or who constantly cross thresholds,[51]
19′ or [who] constantly climb over roof[s],
20′ or who go about in sewage outlets,
21′ or who constantly sit in rubbish dumps.[52]

In the context of sewage outlets and rubbish dumps, it is possible that the imagery of the demon going in and out of houses, particularly crossing their thresholds, is intended to represent the threat of waste, especially dirty water building up in the street, encroaching into people's homes and threatening the health of the inhabitants.

3 Demons as pollution

The passage cited above comes from the eleventh tablet of Udug-ḫul, also known as Marduk's Address to the Demons. It consists of a long Akkadian incantation in which Asalluḫi-Marduk addresses the demons directly, in the latter half describing their nature and behavior. Another passage from this part of Marduk's Address is similar to that previously cited but has various difficulties of interpretation, which can now be partly resolved in the context of the preceding discussion. The passage describes various actions performed by and against the demons (UH XI 70′–82′):

70′ *lu-u*$_2$ *ša*$_2$ *dūrānī*(bad$_3$)^{meš} ⸢*ta*⸣*-at-ta-nab-lak-ka-*⸢*tu*⸣
71′ [*lu-u*$_2$] ⸢*ša*$_2$⸣ *šur-ša*$_2$*-*⸢*ra*⸣*-a-*⸢*ta*⸣ (?) *ta-at-ta-na-*⸢*at*⸣*-ba-ku*
72′ [*lu*]*-*⸢*u*⸣ *ša*$_2$ *ina a-sur-re-e tattanaššaba*(dur$_2$.dur$_2$)^{ba}
73′ ⸢*lu*⸣*-u ša*$_2$ *īkī*(e)^{meš} *te-eš-te-ne*$_2$*-ʾi-i-ri*
74′ *lu-u ša*$_2$ *palgī*(pa$_5$)^{meš} *ta-aš-ta-na-aḫ-ḫi-*⸢*ṭa?*⸣
75′ *lu-u ša*$_2$ *ina ni-gi-iṣ-ṣa-a-ti taḫ-te-ne*$_2$*-es-sa-a*
76′ *lu-u ša*$_2$ *a-na nāri*(id$_2$) *kul-lu-ma-tu-nu*
77′ *lu-u ša*$_2$ *a-na nāri*(id$_2$) *ṭa-ab-ḫa-tu-nu*
78′ *lu-u* ⸢*ša*$_2$⸣ ⸢*ana*⸣ *nāri*(id$_2$) *pur-ru-sa-tu-nu*
79′ ⸢*lu*⸣*-u ša*$_2$ *ina nāri*(id$_2$) *tar-ta-na-aḫ-ḫi-ṣa*
80′ *lu-u ša*$_2$ *ina nāri*(id$_2$) *kīma*(gin$_7$) *a-mi-ra-nu ta-aṣ-ṣa-nun-du*
81′ ⸢*lu*⸣*-u ša*$_2$ *ina nāri*(id$_2$) *ta-aṣ-ṣa-nun-du*
82′ *lu-u ša*$_2$ *ina* ^{giš}*qīšāti*(tir)^{meš} *tattanallaku*(du.du)^{ku}
70′ Whether (you are ones) who constantly climb over the city walls,
71′ [or] who are constantly poured out . . . (?),
72′ [or] who constantly sit in the sewage outlet,
73′ or who constantly cross ditches,
74′ or who constantly jump over canals,
75′ or who constantly hide in cracks,
76′ or who are displayed for the river,

50 Scurlock 2006: 491, No. 206 3: . . . ⸢*eṭemmu*(gidim) *mê*(a)⸣ *ina ramāki*(tu$_5$) ⸢*iṣbat*(dib)⸣*-su ana napšāti*(zi)^{meš}*-šu*$_2$ *la*$_3$ *kurê*(lugud$_2$.⸢da⸣) " . . . A ghost seized him while he was bathing (in) water. In order that his breaths not be short: (ritual instructions follow)".

51 On the meaning of the verb *šaʾāru/šeʾēru*, see Schwemer 2003.

52 Composite text based on the edition of the electronic Babylonian Library (www.ebl.lmu.de/corpus/L/3/3, accessed 25/01/2023), with additions and corrections to Geller 2016: 368–369, II 17–21. Translation by the author.

77′ or who are slaughtered for the river,
78′ or who are divided up for the river,
79′ or who constantly flood / bathe in the river,
80′ or who prowl in the river like floodwater,
81′ or who prowl in the river,
82′ or who constantly walk about in the forest.[53]

In spite of this passage's many philological difficulties, it is clear that it concerns demons in the context of sewage and various watercourses. The first and last lines included above demonstrate some of the structural motivations of this part of the incantation. It is significant that this passage about waste and rivers is situated between descriptions of demons prowling about the city streets and then in the forest and the steppe. With human settlements encroaching upon the natural environment as well as dangers from the steppe invading the city, the threats represented by both human waste and demons entering rivers effectively transgress the boundary between the city and the steppe. The interpretation that one embodies the other, however, relies on resolving some of the passage's difficulties, which will be addressed in the following commentary.

Since the demons are being addressed directly, we would expect second-person plural verb forms throughout the passage, and indeed lines 76′–78′ contain unproblematic second-person masculine plural stative forms. However, the situation with the remaining finite verbs is not so straightforward, with many of the final vowels written with *-u* instead of the expected *-ā* of the second-person plural suffix. While these spellings could be explained as subjunctive and ventive suffixes on second-person singular verbs, this would not account for a sudden change to the second-person plural in the stative forms, so it is probably best to follow previous translators in interpreting all of the verbs as plural forms, even if this does not fully account for the various spellings.[54] I will now discuss individual lines in more depth.

71′) Another frustrating problem with this passage is the question of what is represented by the writing *šur-ša-ra-ta*. One possibility is to read sur *ša ra-ta*, i.e. *sūru ša rāta* 'ditch of the drainage channel', which would certainly bear a semantic relation to the *asurrû* in the following line.[55] The spelling of the genitive with *-a* remains problematic, however, as does the phrase's exact relationship to the verb with no preposition governing it ('who are constantly poured out *into* the ditch of the drainage channel'?).

Alternatively, the writing may represent a corruption of a phonetically similarly word, such as *šuršurrātu*. Taking it as *šuršurrātu* 'chains' seems unlikely given both the sense of the passage and the fact that this form is otherwise only attested in the Middle Assyrian period.[56] On the other hand, a feminine plural of the word *šuršurru* presents an interesting possibility. The term *šuršurru* is usually understood to refer to a type of fruit, due to it occurring as a variant of *šuršašnu* (= *nurmû* 'pomegranate') in a witness to the lexical composition *Malku* = *šarru* and together with *ḫinzurru* 'apple' in a hymn to Nabû.[57] In a text concerning medical conditions of the eyes (BAM 510), the term occurs among things that might figuratively cause irritation in the eye, including other common sources of ritual contamination (iv 34–36): . . . *am-mi-ni ta-aš-ša-ni ḫa-*⸢*ma*⸣ / *ḫa-an-d*[*a-bi-l*]*u*$^{?}$ *šu-ur-šu-ra e-lap*$^{?}$*-pa-a ša nāri*(id$_2$) *ina sūqāti*(sila)^{meš} *kir-ba-ni* / *ina tub-k*[*in*$_2$*-na*]-⸢*a*⸣*-te ḫu-ṣa-a-ba am-mi-ni taš-ša-ni* . . . "Why are you carrying chaff, *ḫandabillu-pebbles*, *šuršurru*, algae of the river? In the street, a clod of earth, in the rubbish dumps, leavings (lit. splinters), why are you carrying (them)?"[58] The context of this passage suggests that *šuršurru* may represent a type of algae or other river plant (perhaps resembling a pomegranate or apple) that was as dangerous as the contagious material being carried away from the rubbish dumps, perhaps also by flowing water. The evidence is far from conclusive, but identifying *šuršurrātu* in the Udug-ḫul passage as a harmful algae would be appropriate, since it is associated with demons that were a dangerous presence in rivers and canals.

---

53 Composite text based on the edition of the electronic Babylonian Library (www.ebl.lmu.de/corpus/L/3/3, accessed 25/01/2023), with additions and corrections to Geller 2016: 380–382, II 70–80. Translation by the author.

54 E.g. Geller 2016: 380–382; Foster 2005: 956–957 (different but parallel passage).

55 For *sūru*, see CAD S 415 (although note that the usual logographic spelling is sur$_3$ rather than sur$_1$); for *rāṭ/tu*, see CAD R 219–220.

56 CAD Š/3 366.

57 CAD Š/3 366, with references.

58 The edition and translation here follow that of Geller and Panayotov 2020: 104–15, 187′–189′, but see also Collins 1999: 216–218 and Zomer 2023: 68.

Along similar lines, the writing may be a corruption of the term *šūšurātu* 'sweepings', which also fits with the semantic context here, and appears alongside the term *asurrû* in a passage from *Maqlû*, in which the patient describes how the witches might be disposed of (II 179–180): *ki-ma mê*(a)^{meš} *mu-sa-a-ti a-sur-ra-a u$_2$-ma-al-la-šu$_2$-nu-ti / ki-ma šu-*⸢*šu*⸣*-rat bīti*(e$_2$) *ana bābi*(ka$_2$) *a-na-as-suk-šu$_2$-nu-*⸢*ti*⸣ "Like wash-water I am filling the sewage outlet with them, like sweepings of the house I am removing them through the doorway". If this was the term intended here, then the demons would be represented as another form of household waste alongside their association with sewage, both of which eventually find their way into canals and rivers. However, none of these suggestions resolves the problem of the word's function in the sentence and relationship to the verb: if algae or sweepings are meant they could be in apposition with the demons as subject of the verb (i.e. "who are constantly poured out *as* algae/sweepings"), thus effectively identifying one with the other, but this also does not fully explain the spelling.

72′) This line is similar to one in another previously discussed passage (UH XI 21′), but here the demons are sitting or dwelling (*wašābu*) not in rubbish dumps but in sewage outlets, both well established as haunts of demons.

73′) Geller emends the object in this line to *bītāti*(e$_2$$^!$)^{meš} 'houses' (possibly on the basis of the preceding lines UH XI 17′–18′),[59] but retaining *īkī*(e)^{meš} 'ditches' makes more sense in this context. The reference to ditches further supports the suggestion that the verb *še'ēru* primarily means 'cross over', especially with the action described in the following line.

74′) With the references to *īku* 'ditch' in the preceding line and *palgu* '(irrigation) canal' in this line, the passage seems to be tracing the demons' (and perhaps also the waste's) journey from urban wastewater outlets, via agricultural water channels, to the canals and rivers that connected the world settled by humans to the steppe beyond. The verb *šaḫāṭu* 'jump' with a direct object suggests 'jump over', an action that is associated with canals in other texts,[60] reflecting the demons' ability to cross environmental boundaries to access their victims as well as their association with watercourses. It possibly also plays on the homophonous verb *šaḫāt/ṭu* 'wash/strip off',[61] in parallel with the verb *raḫāṣu* 'wash' later (79′), suggesting that the demons are washing off their own impurities in the canals and rivers, to the disadvantage of any humans also using them for washing, irrigation, or drinking.

75′) In another part of the previously discussed passages from Saĝ-ba (I 117–118) and ASKT 11 (184–185), the term *nigiṣṣu* seems to refer to cracks in the fabric of the victim's house, and in both instances the word is preceded by references to holes (ḫabrud // *ḫurru*). In this context, it perhaps refers to cracks in dried mud on the banks of canals and rivers, which would be an appropriate hiding place for demons. Similarly, the illness *maškadu*, which causes muscle and joint pain in humans and could be contracted from livestock,[62] is described in an Old Babylonian incantation lurking in a pit (*šitpum*) and in the footprint of an ox (*kibis alpim*),[63] both of which are also holes or depression in the ground.

76′–78′) In these lines the string of finite verbs is interrupted by three 2mp stative forms, and surprisingly the verbs used give the impression that the demon are being offered in sacrifice to the river. The verb *kullumu* 'make visible, show, display' is very rarely used in the D-stem to refer to offerings made to gods,[64] but this sense would correspond to that of the more common cognate nouns *taklīmu* and *taklimtu*, which can both refer to types of funerary offering.[65] Although unusual, the sense of a cultic display or offering for *kullumu* is strengthened by the following verbs. The verb *tabāḫu* is the standard term for slaughtering an animal, often as a sacrifice.[66] The D-stem of *parāsu* means to 'divide', in the sense of either dismembering or apportioning something, both of which would be appropriate in the context of sacrifice and offering. It seems unlikely that anyone would want or be able to sacrifice a demon to the divine river, so these lines must describe a more prosaic form of giving a demon, or at least some sort of impurity conceptualized as a

59 Geller 2016: 380.

60 E.g. Lambert 1960: 253, 8–9: *tu-uš-te-gir / pal-ga ul ta-ša$_2$-ḫi-iṭ* "You are twisted, you cannot jump over a canal".

61 See now Ambos 2024 for the case that the two verbs usually separated by the dictionaries, *šaḫātu* 'wash off' and *šaḫāṭu* 'strip off', are probably one and the same, with the key difference being that washing can transfer impurities to another medium, as I suggest the demons are doing here.

62 See e.g. Wasserman 2012, Arbøll 2018.

63 Collins 1999: 234, 10–11.

64 Two examples are cited in CAD K 523.

65 Cf. CAD T 80–81.

66 Cf. CAD Ṭ 1–4.

demon, to the river. Perhaps, therefore, it is euphemistically describing the dumping of household waste into a river, or how it makes its own way from the sewage outlet to the river.

79′–81′) In these lines the demons now appear to be in the river, prowling and washing themselves, and they are compared to floodwater. The verb *raḫāṣu* seems to have a basic meaning of flushing or flooding with water, giving rise to two specific senses:[67] 'overwhelm', used primarily of the storm god Adad inundating fields and striking down people and animals;[68] and 'wash' or 'rinse', in the sense of flushing with water for the purpose of ritual or medical cleansing.[69] Again, the double meaning is probably intentional here: the demons are like dirty water flooding into rivers (and are indeed described as a flood in the following line), and are also rinsing themselves of their own impurities in the river, and thus polluting the water. The term *amirānu* refers specifically to standing water, either in a swamp or left over after a flood,[70] which is a fitting comparison here, as this would have been a particularly fetid and dangerous form of water.

The imagery in this passage begins with a reference to the sewage outlet and perhaps other waste, and transitions from urban wastewater channels, via agricultural irrigation canals, to the natural watercourses flowing around and away from human habitation. It therefore seems to be describing the process of waste running off into rivers, or being dumped directly into rivers, by conceptualizing it in terms of demons lurking around canals, being offered in sacrifice to the river, and swimming about and washing in the water. Rivers, although far from ideal due to their location and the presence of pollution, presumably served as sources of water for various uses, including cooking, washing, irrigation, and industrial uses, if not for drinking water.[71] Any contamination of rivers was therefore to be avoided: for example, urinating and spitting into rivers were apparently proscribed.[72] There is some evidence from medical texts for an awareness of water-borne diseases,[73] but it is unlikely that a distinction could have been made between those caused by pollutants and other vectors like insects, amoebae, or venomous fish. The danger to health posed by water from polluted rivers was therefore known but, without germ theory, this threat had to be expressed in terms of the actions of demons, with the above passage perhaps also serving as a warning against disposing of waste in rivers. This does not mean, however, that the audience of such incantations had an understanding of pollution similar to ours. Rivers were divine, emanating from the underground freshwater Apsû and having special purifying abilities, and this is also why they served as an ideal place for dumping contaminated materials. While there was a recognition of the danger posed by river pollutants, this was presumably conceived in terms of the sort of cultic contamination associated with other ritual materials and not in terms of epidemiology, while the illnesses that they caused were, like many other illnesses, attributed to the evil actions of demons.

4 Conclusions

There are many invisible dangers that form an unavoidable part of living in close proximity to other people. Some of these were recognized in Mesopotamia, and various architectural and behavioral measures were taken in an attempt to manage them. However, with limited understanding of the workings of contagious illness, these interventions would have had limited success in reducing illness and death, so these intangible threats were simultaneously confronted

67 These are separated in the CAD (R 69–74), but treated as a single lemma in the AHw (II 942–943).

68 See Schwemer 2001: 63 n. 364, with further references.

69 It is in this sense that the derived noun *marḫaṣu* is used to refer to enemas (cf. Goltz 1974: 79–80).

70 Cf. CAD A/2 63.

71 Wells were apparently relatively rare as a source of drinking water in Mesopotamia (Van de Mieroop 1997: 158–161). Beer may have been drunk as a safer alternative to water: there is evidence for its use as an intoxicant in social contexts, but the alcohol levels in Mesopotamian beer were probably low enough for it to be drunk more regularly (Damerow 2012: 18). In *Ištar's Descent to the Netherworld*, Ereškigal laments the possibility of having to drink turbid water (*mê dalḫūte*) instead of beer (cf. Röllig 1970: 67).

72 *Šurpu* III 63 (Reiner 1958: 21): *ma-mit nāra*(id$_2$) *ša$_2$-a-nu u nāra*(id$_2$) *ka-a-a*<*-u*> "Curse of urinating (into) a river or spitting (into) a river". Van de Mieroop (1997: 160) warns against using this as a source for everyday practice, but spitting in public was certainly dangerous as the saliva could be collected and used for witchcraft (cf. Schwemer 2007: 90–91).

73 There are several references to symptoms associated with bathing in rivers, including fever, bloating, and skin lesions, all of which occur while in the water or shortly after getting out (Scurlock and Andersen 2005: 363–365). The exorcist attributed these symptoms to a *rābiṣu* of the river (Scurlock and Andersen 2005: 365), an epithet also applied to the demon Šulak.

within the framework of a discourse that attributed the causes of many illnesses to demons. Demons could be used to conceptualize seemingly random natural occurrences that threatened the health and wellbeing of humans, including their role in personifying certain illnesses. It appears that demons were also employed to explain and manage the dangers posed by human effluence and household waste. Demons could serve as a way of expressing fears about these dangers, by giving invisible contagions a more concrete and ritually manageable form, and perhaps also as a way of discouraging the careless disposal of waste, something that was a frequent concern for exorcists with their magically contagious waste products. At the same time, if these dangers are attributed to demons, there is little motivation to deal with waste in a way that would effectively reduce the danger to public health (i.e. performing rituals against demons rather than actually keeping water sources clean). The risks and associated illnesses would therefore persist, serving as further proof that powerful malicious demons really were at work. However, by attributing these dangers not to germs, which Mesopotamian medicine did not have the tools to understand, but to demons, which Mesopotamian exorcists already had a well-established framework for dealing with through rituals and incantations, they could at least effectively manage anxieties around one aspect of the 'paradox' of urbanism.

Bibliography

Abou-Assaf et al. 1982 = A. Abou-Assaf, P. Bordreuil, and A. R. Millard, *La Statue de Tell Fekherye et son inscription bilingue assyro-araméenne* (Paris: Editions Recherche sur les civilisations)

Abusch and Schwemer 2011 = T. Abusch and D. Schwemer, *Corpus of Mesopotamian Anti-Witchcraft Rituals, Volume 1*, Ancient Magic and Divination 8/1 (Leiden and Boston: Brill)

Abusch et al. 2020 = T. Abusch, D. Schwemer, M. Luukko and G. van Buylaere, *Corpus of Mesopotamian Anti-Witchcraft Rituals, Volume 3*, Ancient Magic and Divination 8/3 (Leiden and Boston: Brill)

Algaze 2018 = G. Algaze, 'Entropic Cities: The Paradox of Urbanism in Ancient Mesopotamia', *Current Anthropology* 59/1, 23–54

Ambos 2024 = C. Ambos, 'Mesopotamische Abstreif- und Abspülriten: Zur Unterscheidung von šaḫātu ("abspülen") und šaḫātu ("abstreifen")', in: níĝ-ba dub-sar maḫ: Studies on Ebla and the Ancient Near East presented to Amalia Catagnoti, ed. E. Cianfanelli and F. Gori, Documenta Asiana 14 (Rome: Edizioni Quasar), 27–30

Arbøll 2018 = T. P. Arbøll, 'Tracing Mesopotamian Medical Knowledge: A Study of *maškadu* and Related Illnesses', in: *Sources of Evil: Studies in Mesopotamian Exorcistic Lore*, ed. G. Van Buylaere, M. Luukko, D. Schwemer, and A. Mertens-Wagschal, Ancient Magic and Divination 15 (Leiden and Boston: Brill), 261–284

Bácskay 2017 = A. Bácskay, 'The Natural and Supernatural Aspects of Fever in Mesopotamian Medical Texts', in: *Demons and Illness from Antiquity to the Early-Modern Period*, ed. S. Bhayro and C. Rider, Magic and Religious Literature of Late Antiquity 5 (Leiden and Boston: Brill), 39–52

Biggs 1993 = R. D. Biggs, 'Descent of Ištar, line 104', *NABU* 1993/3, 58–59

Borger 1969 = R. Borger, 'Die erste Teiltafel der zi-pà-Beschwörungen (ASKT 11), in: *Lišān mitḫurti, FS Wolfram von Soden*, ed. M. Dietrich and W. Röllig (Neukirchen-Vluyn: Verlag Butzon & Bercker Kevelaer), 1–22

Cavigneaux and Al-Rawi 1993 = A. Cavigneaux and F. Al-Rawi, 'New Sumerian Literary Texts from Tell Haddad (Ancient Meturan): A First Survey', *Iraq* 55, 91–105

Collins 1999 = T. J. Collins, *Natural Illness in Babylonian Medical Incantations* [PhD dissertation, University of Chicago] (Chicago)

Damerow 2012 = P. Damerow, 'Sumerian Beer: The Origins of Brewing Technology in Ancient Mesopotamia', *Cuneiform Digital Library Journal* 2012: 2

Eypper 2016 = S. Eypper, 'Diseases of the Feet in Babylonian-Assyrian Medicine. A Study of Text K. 67+', *Journal des Médecines Cunéiformes* 27, 1–58

Feder 2016 = Y. Feder, 'Defilement, Disgust, and Disease: The Experiential Basis of Hittite and Akkadian Terms for Impurity', *Journal of the American Oriental Society* 136/1, 99–116

Feder 2022 = Y. Feder, *Purity and Pollution in the Hebrew Bible: From Embodied Experience to Moral Metaphor* (Cambridge, New York, Port Melbourne, New Delhi, and Singapore: Cambridge University Press)

Fincke 2013 = J. C. Fincke, '^d*Šaggāšu* ("Murderer"), The Demon from the Steppe', *Bibliotheca Orientalis* 70/1–2, 17–24

Foster 2005 = B. R. Foster, *Before the Muses. An Anthology of Akkadian Literature* [Third edition] (Bethesda: CDL Press)

Freedman 1998 = S. M. Freedman, *If a City is Set on a Height. The Akkadian Omen Series Šumma ālu ina mēlê šakin, Volume 1: Tablets 1–21*, Occasional Publication of the Samuel Noah Kramer Fund 17 (Philadelphia: University of Pennsylvania Museum of Archaeology and Anthropology)

Geller 2016 = M. J. Geller, *Healing Magic and Evil Demons: Canonical Udug-Hul Incantations*, Die babylonisch-assyrische Medizin in Texten und Untersuchungen 8 (Boston and Berlin: De Gruyter)

Geller and Panayotov 2020 = M. J. Geller and S. V. Panayotov, *Mesopotamian Eye Disease Texts: The Nineveh Treatise*, Die babylonisch-assyrische Medizin in Texten und Untersuchungen 10 (Boston and Berlin: De Gruyter)

George 1999 = A. R. George, 'Marc van de Mieroop: *The ancient Mesopotamian city*' [Review], *Bulletin of the School of Oriental and African Studies* 62/3, 550–552

George 2015 = A. R. George, 'On Babylonian Lavatories and Sewers', *Iraq* 72, 75–106

Goltz 1974 = D. Goltz, *Studien zur altorientalischen und griechischen Heilkunde: Therapie, Arneibereitung, Rezeptstruktur* (Wiesbaden: Steiner)

Greenfield and Schafer 1983 = J. C. Greenfield and A. Schafer, *'qlqlt' tubkinnu*, Refuse Tips and Treasure Trove', *Anatolian Studies* 33, 123–129

Hemker 1993 = C. Hemker, *Altorientalische Kanalisation: Untersuchungen zu Be- und Entwässerungsanlagen im mesopotamisch – syrisch – anatolischen Raum*, Abhandlungen der Deutschen-Orient-Gesellschaft 22 (Münster: Asgenda)

Krafeld-Daugherty 1994 = M. Krafeld-Daugherty, *Wohnen im Alten Orient. Eine Untersuchung zur Verwendung von Räumen in altorientalischen Wohnhäusern*, Altertumskunde des Vorderen Orients 3 (Münster: Ugarit-Verlag)

Læssøe 1955 = J. Læssøe, *Studies on the Assyrian ritual and series bît rimki* (Copenhagen: Munksgaard)

Lambert 1954–56 = W. G. Lambert 'An Address of Marduk to the Demons', *Archiv für Orientforschung* 17, 310–321

Lambert 1960 = W. G. Lambert, *Babylonian Wisdom Literature* (Oxford: Oxford University Press)

Lambert 1979 = W. G. Lambert, 'W. von Soden (ed.), *Akkadisches Handwörterbuch: unter Benutzung des lexikalischen Nachlasses von Bruno Meissner (1868–1947)*, Lief. 12, 13 and 14' [Review], *Journal of Semitic Studies* 24/2, 268–273

Maul 1994 = S. M. Maul, *Zukunftsbewältigung: Eine Untersuchung altorientalischen Denkens anhand der babylonisch-assyrischen Löserituale (Namburbi)*, Baghdader Forschungen 18 (Mainz: Verlag Philipp von Zabern)

McMahon 2015 = A. McMahon, 'Waste Management in Early Urban Southern Mesopotamia', in: *Sanitation, Latrines and Intestinal Parasites in Past Populations*, ed. P. D. Mitchell (Farnham and Burlington: Routledge), 19–39

Preusser 1954 = C. Preusser, *Die Wohnhäuser in Assur*, Wissenschaftliche Veröffentlichungen der Deutschen Orient-Gesellschaft 64 (Berlin: Gebr. Mann)

Reiner 1958 = E. Reiner, *Šurpu. A Collection of Sumerian and Akkadian Incantations*, Archiv für Orientforschung Beiheft 11 (Osnabrück: Biblio Verlag)

Reuther 1926 = O. Reuther, *Die Innenstadt von Babylon (Merkes)*, Wissenschaftliche Veröffentlichung der Deutschen Orient-Gesellschaft 47 (Leipzig: J.C. Hinrichs)

Röllig 1970 = W. Röllig, *Das Bier im alten Mesopotamien* (Berlin: Gesellschaft für Geschichte des Brauwesens e.V.)

Schramm 2001 = W. Schramm, *Bann, Bann! Eine sumerisch-akkadische Beschwörungsserie*, Göttinger Arbeitshefte zur altorientalischen Literatur 2 (Göttingen: Seminar für Keilschriftforschung)

Schwemer 2001 = D. Schwemer, *Die Wettergottgestalten Mesopotamiens und Nordsyriens im Zeitalter der Keilschriftkunden. Materialien und Studien nach den schriftlichen Quellen* (Wiesbaden: Harrassowitz)

Schwemer 2003 = D. Schwemer, 'Akkadisch *še'ēru*, *ša'āru*', *NABU* 2003/4, 108

Schwemer 2007 = D. Schwemer, *Abwehrzauber und Behexung: Studien zum Schadenzauberglauben im alten Mesopotamien* (Wiesbaden: Harrassowitz)

Scurlock 2006 = J.-A. Scurlock, *Magico-Medical Means of Treating Ghost-Induced Illnesses in Ancient Mesopotamia*, Ancient Magic and Divination 3 (Leiden and Boston: Brill)

Scurlock and Andersen 2005 = J.-A. Scurlock and B. R. Andersen, *Diagnoses in Assyrian and Babylonian Medicine* (Urbana and Chicago: University of Illinois Press)

Steinert 2014 = U. Steinert, 'City Streets: Reflections on Urban Society in the Cuneiform Sources of the Second and First Millennium BCE', in: *The Fabric of Cities: Aspects of Urbanism, Urban Topography and Society in Mesopotamia, Greece and Rome*, ed. N. N. May and U. Steinert, Culture and History of the Ancient Near East 68 (Leiden and Boston: Brill), 123–169

Stol 1993 = M. Stol, *Epilepsy in Babylonia*, Cuneiform Monographs 2 (Groningen: Styx publications)

Stol 2020 = M. Stol, 'Abusch, T., D. Schwemer, M. Luukko and G. Van Buylaere – Corpus of Mesopotamian Anti-Wticraft Rituals. Volume Three & Van Buylaere, G. and M. Luukko – Corpus of Mesopotamian Anti-Witchcraft Rituals. Volume Four' [Review], *Bibliotheca Orientalis* 77/5–6, 567–573

Tenney 2017 = J. S. Tenney, 'Babylonian Populations, Servility, and Cuneiform Records', *Journal of the Economic and Social History of the Orient* 60, 715–787

Van Buylaere and Luukko 2020 = G. van Buylaere and M. Luukko, *Corpus of Mesopotamian Anti-Witchcraft Rituals, Volume 4, Glossaries and Indices*, Ancient Magic and Divination 8/4 (Leiden and Boston: Brill)

Van de Mieroop 1997 = M. van de Mieroop, *The Ancient Mesopotamian City* (Oxford: Oxford University Press)

Van der Toorn 1985 = K. van der Toorn, *Sin and Sanction in Israel and Mesopotamia: A Comparative Study* (Assen and Maastricht: Van Gorcum)

Wasserman 2012 = N. Wasserman, '*Maškadum* and Other Zoonotic Diseases in Medical and Literary Akkadian Sources', *Bibliotheca Orientalis* 69/5–6, 426–436.

Welton 2020 = R. Welton, *'He is a Glutton and a Drunkard': Deviant Consumption in Hebrew Bible*, Biblical Interpretation Series 183 (Leiden and Boston: Brill)

Wiggermann 1992 = F. A. M. Wiggermann, *Mesopotamian Protective Spirits: The Ritual Texts*, Cuneiform Monographs 1 (Grongingen: Styx)

Zomer 2023 = E. Zomer, 'Negotiating with Evil: The Rhetorical Strategy of *epiplexis* in Mesopotamian Magic', in: *Legitimising Magic: Strategies and Practices in Ancient Mesopotamia*, ed. N. P. Heeßel and E. Zomer, Ancient Magic and Divination 21 (Leiden and Boston: Brill), 56–76

Marta Iommelli

"The Asakku-demon Who Rolls in on the Earth Like a Storm": Analyzing Diseases That Attack Humans and Cattle According to the Mesopotamian Perspective

In ancient Mesopotamia, the treatment of infections and other diseases drew on medical knowledge as well as on religious beliefs and magical interventions. The ancient understanding of the relationship between cause and symptom encompassed both the physical and the supernatural, such a perspective, alien to our modern interpretative model, has led modern scholars to reflect on ancient mind, society and science in their work on these sources. In this framework, one of the most complex issues is the relationship between humans and animals stricken by diseases that Mesopotamian healers believed affected both equally. The animals which were considered to share diseases with humans are mostly mammals, including cattle, small ruminants, horses, and dogs

This issue has already been explored in several contributions discussing the concept of zoonosis and some diseases listed in Mesopotamian therapeutic documentation that could be considered as such.[1] However, the transmission of pathological states from humans to animals in Mesopotamian sources is a topic that deserves further exploration and the application of new forms of investigation that do not rely solely on the technique of retrospective diagnosis – i.e. the identification of diseases based on the description of symptoms listed in Mesopotamian medical literature – but rather frame this issue within an epistemological perspective.[2]

To accomplish this objective, it was necessary to examine the matter in a wider context. Section 1 investigates whether Mesopotamian society had an understanding of contagion and zoonosis. To achieve this, we analyze various archival materials, such as letters, legal codes, technical therapeutic literature, and lexical lists. Sections 2 and 3 examine two case studies of demons found in healing incantations and rituals. These entities, namely Samana and Asakku, as depicted in Mesopotamian sources, appear linked to two highly contagious infectious diseases affecting both humans and animals, particularly livestock. Section 4 discusses the conclusions drawn from the analysis.

1 The Concept of Zoonosis

According to the modern biomedical perspective, zoonoses are infections or diseases that can be transmitted directly or indirectly between animals and humans. The study of zoonotic diseases in historical records provides valuable insights into the relationships between human societies, domestic animals and wildlife. It also enhances our understanding of the environmental and socio-cultural factors that influenced disease transmission, and clarifies how ancient societies perceived and managed the health risks associated with close contact with animals.

However, before discussing zoonotic diseases, it is important to investigate whether people in Mesopotamia were aware of the existence of such diseases and whether they believed that diseases could be transmitted through contact or proximity between humans and animals. Some clues can be found in the corpus of Tell el-Amarna, where on several

1 Kämmerer 1995; Yuhong 2001; Wasserman 2012; Arbøll 2021b. For general discussion about contagion and infections, see also Nutton 2000.
2 For a discussion on the merits and limitations of retrospective diagnosis, refer to Heeßel 2004.

Note: The title of this paper is taken from UH III 2. For the translation, see Geller 2016: 90. I would like to express my gratitude to Troels P. Arbøll for inviting me to participate in the conference titled "Infecting the Ancient Mesopotamian Cosmos" held at Oxford, from which this paper originates. His valuable insights and constructive feedback, along with the contributions of Simonetta Graziani, Gian Pietro Basello, and Markham Geller, have been instrumental in shaping this paper. The responsibility for the ideas expressed here, as well as any mistakes, is entirely my own. Additionally, I would like to express my appreciation to all conference participants for their stimulating discussions and supportive feedback.

Marta Iommelli, University of Naples "L' Orientale"

 | https://doi.org/10.1515/9783112238622-003

occasions the occurrence of an epidemic[3] striking the country is mentioned in the letters. Thanks to these references found in the epistolary documentation[4] it is possible to determine the extent of the awareness about how the infections worked and the strategies adopted to cope with them (such as quarantine). It is clear, for example, that proximity is recognized as one of the possible causes of the spreading of diseases and that the fear of contagion blocked the normal trade flow and prevented the movement of goods and military troops.

Besides Amarna, an outstanding part of the documentation comes from Mari, where clues regarding epidemics,[5] infectious diseases, and the countermeasures adopted to prevent their spread throughout the kingdom are recorded in letters.[6] A striking example is provided by a letter[7] from Ašqudum to Zimri-Lim where an epidemic that had hit the upper district is mentioned and the precautionary measures adopted (the quarantine) are clearly stated:

> "The god is striking in the upper district, so I without delay took a bypass. Furthermore, my lord should give orders that inhabitants of the towns, as soon as they have been 'touched', must not enter into 'untouched' towns. It is to be feared that they will 'touch' all the country. (. . .) My lord should stop at Terqa and he must not go to Saggarâtum. That land is 'touched'."[8]

It is worth mentioning that not just epidemics but also contagious diseases were reported in Mari's letters. The places where illnesses proliferated mostly were the ones where people spent time close to each other, such as the palace and in particular the harem of the king. Insight about this condition is given by a letter written from Zimri-Lim to Šibtu[9] about Nanna, a woman of the entourage of the king suffering from a contagious disease (*simmum*). The prevention measures listed in the following example clearly show awareness of the transmission of this disease by proximity or contact:

> "[To] Šibtu, thus speaks your lord. I have learned that Nanna is ill with a disease: so far, she is in her palace and many women mingle with her. Now give inflexible orders: that no one drink from the cup where she drank, that no one sit on the chair where she sat and that no one lie down in the bed where she lay and let her refrain from mingling with many women! That disease is contagious (*muštaḫḫizu*)."[10]

A further source highlighting awareness of contagion in Mesopotamia are spells and rituals. One of many examples comes from the incantation series *Šurpu*, quoted below. It is particularly remarkable for the similarities with the letter mentioned above, as it is also an expression of the belief that the purity of a person can be affected by direct contact with someone who is impure, an "accursed" person *tamû*.[11] In the mindset of Mesopotamians, the concept of purity, or better the concept of impurity, is treated as an illness (and perhaps *vice versa*), and it is ruled by the mechanism of contagion: "He slept in the bed of an 'accursed' person (*tamû*), he sat on the chair of an 'accursed' person, he ate at the table of an 'accursed' person, he drank from the cup of an 'accursed' person".[12]

---

3 In this documentation the word for plague, epidemic or pestilence is *mūtānu* (written syllabically or BA.ÚŠ) as in EA 96 and EA 362 (cf. CAD M2: 296 "epidemic, pestilence, plague"). Sometimes epidemics are simply described as the "Hand of Nergal" (as in EA 35).

4 See letters EA 35, 96, and 362.

5 In this documentation the words for epidemics are *ukulti ilim* "devouring by god" and again *mūtānu*. A people or a city struck by the epidemic is *lapit* "touched".

6 See ARM 26/1 no. 17; ARM 26/1 no. 259; AbB 2 no. 118; ARM 5 no. 87.

7 ARM 26/1 no. 17.

8 ARM 26/1 no. 17 rev. 20–30. For translation, see Durand 1988: 127–128 (English translation is made by the author). The Akkadian word is *laptum*, which Durand 1988: 127 translate as "contaminés". I have opted for the translation "touched" in order to uphold a higher degree of fidelity to the original text.

9 ARM 10 no. 129.

10 ARM 10 no. 129 obv. 1–10. For translation, see Dossin 1978: 189 (English translation is made by the author). For the reading Nanna over Nanname, see the edition on Archibab no. 8685. For the term *muštaḫḫizu*, see CAD M 2: 283; Arbøll 2024: 18 n. 40 with further discussion and references.

11 See Guichard and Marti 2013: 89. For discussion about the term *tamû*, see Guichard and Marti 2013: 89 n. 184, which they translate *tamû* as "damned".

12 See Reiner 1958: 16 = *Šurpu* II lines 100–103. For the discussion about the spread of impurity, see Guichard and Marti 2013: 88–89. For a broader perspective of the concept of purity and impurity in Mesopotamia and ancient Near East, see Feder 2016 and 2022 and Frevel and Nihan 2013.

Contagion by proximity or contact has also been observed among animals. The series Udug-ḫul contains several references to demons attacking and slaughtering animals,[13] emphasizing that the attacks occur in the pen.[14] In the Laws of Hammurabi (§249 and §266) if an animal is killed by the attack of a god (most likely an illness)[15] the herdsman is considered innocent and is discharged from duty to refund the owner. The fact that in §266 it is made explicit that the attack of the god can take place in the pen is probably due to the assumption that this was a place where diseases proliferated mostly. This was possibly due to the close proximity among animals and contact with their excrements, as is best clarified in §163 of the ancient legal code known as the Hittite Laws, dating from c. 1650-1500 BCE and preserved on a number of cuneiform tablets found at Hattusa:[16]

> "If anyone's animals are smitten (with disease) by a God (*šiuniaḫta*), and (the owner) purifies them (*parkunuzi*) and drives them off, but he places the refuse on the scrap-pile, but he does not tell his companion and his companion does not know, so that he drives his cattle (there) and they die, there is restitution."[17]

The spread of infection in an animal pen clearly preoccupied the inhabitants of Mesopotamia, as shown in catalogues of healing texts, such as the AMC and relevant sections of KAR 44:

> *šúm-mu* ANŠE.KUR.RA.MEŠ *ina tar-*[*ba-ṣi* . . . T]UR$^?$ BAD-*a-nu* G[ÁL.MEŠ][18]
> If the horses in the stable [. . . are] reduced (and) there [is] an epidemic . . .

> TÙR ÁB GU$_4$.ḪI.A *u* U$_8$.UDU.ḪI.A ANŠE.KUR.RA SIKIL.E.DÈ[19]
> (Rituals) to purify the pen(s) of cattle, flocks and horse.

Unfortunately, medical texts seldom describe the symptoms of pathogens that affect animals.

A rare exception is represented by medical prescriptions that mention pharmacological remedies, mainly based on plant substances, for the treatment of colic in horses (*kīs libbi*), to be administered through the nostrils.[20]

To the best of my knowledge, except for a series of disease names that could affect sheep mentioned in the lexical list Ur$_5$-ra = *ḫubullû* and quoted below in this section, there are no descriptions of symptoms or pathologies that specifically affect cattle or flocks in medical texts. The reason for this disparity is most likely due to the great value of horses compared to cows and sheep, for which a different estimate of the cost/benefit ratio was made. In the case of the latter, rather than opting for pharmacological treatment that certainly would have led to greater costs, a premature and certainly cheaper solution may have been preferred, namely slaughtering the animal.[21] It is different when it comes to surgery which was performed on asses and oxen for one-sixth of a shekel, as attested in the Laws of Hammurabi (§224 and §225). The reason could possibly be that, as also occurs at modern-day farms, a simple surgery was preferred to the more complex and time-consuming pharmacological treatment.

Nevertheless, people in Mesopotamia were aware of the various diseases affecting animals. These ailments were a concern both from an economic point of view and for sanitary reasons. The following letter from Mari provides insight:

> "Say to my Lord, thus says Yaqqim-Addu, your servant:
>
> A fattened ox of the first quality (GU$_4$ NIGA SAG), intended for an offering-*igisûm* had become very fat (*ma-di-iš ik-bi-ir-ma*) and it is choking (*i-ḫa-aš*)[22] and does not want to receive any more food.

13 See UH IV 35 and VII 81–82 edited in Geller 2016.
14 See e.g. Arbøll 2021b: 29–30.
15 For a discussion about the connection between diseases and gods, refer to Heeßel 2007.
16 For an edition of this text refer to Hoffner 1997.
17 Feder 2016: 109; Hoffner 1997: 131, §163/48.
18 AMC line 121, edited by Seinert *et al.* 2018: 218.
19 KAR 44 rev. 24, edited by Geller 2018: 299.
20 See Scurlock 2014: 499, BAM 159 col. v 33–47; Stadhouders 2012: 3, *Šammu šikinšu* Text I § 15 and Stadhouders 2012:12, Text IIIa § 11; Arbøll 2021a: 329–330, RA 15 pl. 79 rev. 4–8.
21 See as an example ARM 27 no. 131 obv. 7–11. In this letter a previous message written by the king Zimri-Lim is reported. Here the king ordered the slaughter of an ill ox for saving at least the meat.
22 For the translation and discussion of the verb *ḫâšu(m)* in this letter, see Heimpel 1996: 40–41.

> In fact, this beef should not be left without care and its meat should lose its quality. My Lord would have to write to me so that I could have this ox loaded and shipped.
>
> In addition, it is feared that in the middle of the trip, this ox will continue to choke. It is therefore necessary for my Lord to send me a cook ([lú]MUḪALDIM/*nuḫatimmu*) so that he can "cut the throat" of this animal (*na-pí-iš-ti* GU_4 *ša-a-tu ú-ta-ar-ru-ma*)[23] and that its meat can enter the palace.
>
> On the other hand, my Lord should not say: "This ox is seized by the *Aḫḫāzu*-demon" (GU_4 *šu-ú a-ḫa-zu-um a-ḫa-am-*[*m*]*a*).[24] I had this ox presented (to the divinity) by Aḫum himself, at my side, and I sent to my Lord his diagnosis (*ta-ḫi-it-ta-šu*)."[25]

Unlike medical texts, which often lack information on animal symptoms, epistolary records can provide some clues. The symptom described in the aforementioned letter is conveyed through the verb *ḫâšu*, which can be translated as either vomiting[26] or, more accurately, choking.[27] This is because ruminants have three forestomachs and are therefore unable to vomit.

This condition is most likely linked to a sickness that affected cattle being exceedingly fattened, as recorded in three additional letters from the royal archives of Mari.[28] Moreover, the servant Yaqqim-Addu reassures Zimri-Lim that he should not fear that "this ox is seized by the *Aḫḫāzu*-demon".[29] The name of the demon corresponds to a human disease well known from medical texts. Various studies have identified it as jaundice, which is usually caused by infection producing several symptoms, including a yellow discoloration of the skin.[30] The given text suggests that *ḫâšu*-chocking is not a significant issue, except for the need to slaughter the animal earlier. However, *aḫḫāzu* appears to be a more severe problem. The affected cow required examination, and a report (*taḫittu*)[31] had to be submitted to the king.

The Old Babylonian epistolary documentation reveals a familiarity with symptoms of diseases affecting livestock and suggests that specialists conducted checks. Furthermore, the mention of *aḫḫāzu*, which is well-known in human medical texts, demonstrates that the same demon or disease could attack both humans and animals. This is seen in the case of horse colic (*kīs libbi*) and cases of rabies, suggesting that the ancient Mesopotamians believed in a common vulnerability of humans and animals to demonic attacks.[32] Even though the healing specialists recognized that the same agent could cause diseases in both humans and animals,[33] they lacked the technical knowledge to determine whether the diseases were the same according to a modern perspective.

In veterinary diagnosis, healers could only rely on symptoms identifiable through external examination or general manifestation of pain. However, based on the available records, there is no written evidence indicating a direct correlation between the symptoms observed in animals and those documented in human diseases. Nevertheless, several diseases that affect humans have the same names as those that affect animals. The lexical list Ur_5-ra = *ḫubullû* includes a section on domestic animals,[34] specifically sheep, and reports various sicknesses that can affect them:

> UDU.[SA.A]D.NIM II[35] *sa-ma-nu*
> UDU.[SA.A]D.NIM II *ra-pa-du*[36]

23 For the translation *napištam turrum* "cut the throat", see Birot 1993: 217 n. c and Heimpel 1996: 40.

24 The transliteration *a-ḫa-am-*[*m*]*a* is taken from the online version of the text, see <https://www.archibab.fr/T8380> (accessed 18/10/2024).

25 ARM 14 no. 5; for translation and commentary, see Durand 2000: 117–119.

26 Durand 2000: 118.

27 Heimpel 1996.

28 ARM 13 no. 25; ARM 14 no. 6; ARM 27 no. 131.

29 ARM 14 no. 5 rev. 21–22.

30 See Scurlock and Andersen 2005: 138–140.

31 In CAD T: 57–58, *ta'ittu* (*taḫḫittu*) is translated as "information, notification". For the translation of this word as "report", see CAD H: 159 (root *ḫ'ṭ* = *ḫâṭu*). For further discussion, see Durand 2000: 119.

32 For a study of rabies in Mesopotamia, see Yuhong 2001.

33 Arbøll 2021a: 87–90.

34 See Oppenheim and Hartman 1945.

35 II represents the symbol MIN, which means "ditto", as in the repetition of the word above, specifically *im-me-ri* = *immeru* meaning "sheep".

36 The *rapādu*-disease, whose name is taken from the verb *rapādu* "to wander, to roam" (CAD R: 147), features abnormal behavior with shouting and wandering, mostly associated with some kind of trauma. See also Scurlock and Andersen 2005: 350. Additionally, *rapādu* is a phytonym of a plant associated with insanity, but also used to induce inebriation, see Stol, 2017: 374.

UDU.[SA.A]D.GAL II *šá-áš-šá-ṭu*[37]
UDU.[SA.A]D.GAL II *ra-pa-du*[38]

The co-occurrence of pathologies with the same names as human diseases in a specific animal species suggests that these symptoms were observed in those animals.

Mesopotamian specialists used the same names to identify diseases affecting both humans and animals, implying that these illnesses were considered identical and possibly shared a common symptomatology.[39] Therefore, it is likely that, at least from the Mesopotamian perspective, the agent responsible for the illnesses was the same. Despite the absence of explicit evidence within the texts indicating an ancient understanding of disease transmission between animals and humans (or *vice versa*), the awareness of contagion within Mesopotamia, along with the observation that illnesses affecting both humans and animals shared identical names, and the practice of conducting health checks on animals prior to slaughter, collectively suggest that there was at least a cognizance of the risks associated with zoonosis.

2 The Samana-Demon

The *samānu*-disease is connected with the Samana-demon,[40] which is described in the incantations texts as a *Mischwesen* having the mouth of a lion, the teeth of a dragon, the claws on an eagle and the tail of a scorpion.[41] Samana is also associated with the name of a pest affecting barley,[42] an insect,[43] and a kermes worm.[44]

In addition to the lexical list Ur$_5$-ra = *ḫubullû* quoted in Section 1 above, which records the *samānu*-disease affecting sheep, there are some references of medical interest regarding the Samana-demon attacking livestock that can be traced in incantation texts, published by I. L. Finkel.[45] These texts are an important source for understanding the conceptualization of this demon and disease.

The Samana-demon was believed to afflict several types of animals, including sheep,[46] oxen,[47] donkeys,[48] and stags.[49] In addition, the sources provide clues as to which parts of the animal's body were affected by the disease:

It affects the ox in its palate(?) (gu$_4$-e a-ub<-ba> ba-ni-ba)[50]
It affects the sheep in its hoof (udu umbin-ba ba-ni-ba)
It affects the donkey in its ear (anše geštug-ba ba-ni-ba)
It affects the stag in its horn (dàra-maš (?) si-ba ba-ni-ba)[51]

37 *Šaššaṭu* is a disease that affects the patients with muscle jerking, spasms, and rigidity. It was identified as tetanus by Scurlock and Andersen 2005: 66–68. Arbøll 2018 suggests instead the possibility that *šaššaṭu* represented the final stage of an illness, with preceding stages being *maškadu* and *sagallu*.

38 Ur$_5$-ra XIII 57–60 (MSL 8/1: 12).

39 A critical voice might say that lexical lists, such as Ur$_5$-ra = *ḫubullû*, is not necessarily a specialist text as it was used to train everyone in writing. But it was certainly also known by scholars such as Kiṣir-Aššur, see Arbøll 2021a: 21.

40 Böck 2014: 55, 98–99. For a comprehensive overview of the documentation pertaining to Samana as an illness in humans, animals, and plants, see Stol 2006–08.

41 Finkel 1998: 72–74, AO 11276 obv. 2–4.

42 Interpreted as an ergot-like blight on grain (see CAD S: 112), though the translation was rejected by R. D. Biggs who wrote: "In my opinion, all passages connected with barley refer to an insect or a field pest and do not suggest identification with ergot - the harmful effects of which were not known until modern times" (Biggs 1991: 20).

43 KAR 181 rev. 6: [*s*]*a-ma-*[*nu*] *ḫa-líp sa-an-ti* [*e-p*]*iš* [*me*]*-sír-šú ša uqnâ* [*kīma*] *kakkabi i-ṣa-ri-iḫ*, "*Samānu* ist (in einem Mantel) von Rotstein gekleidet, verfertigt ist sein Gürtel aus Blaustein, wie ein Stern funkelt er" (MSL 2: 114).

44 CAD T: 467, citing the third tablet of Uruanna line 237.

45 See Finkel 1998.

46 Finkel 1998: 79–80, HS 1555+1587 rev. 15; 82–83, A 7885 rev. 18; ibid. 88, SU.51/128+ line 14.

47 Finkel 1998: 79–80, HS 1555+1587 rev. 14; ibid.: 82–83, A 7885 rev. 18; ibid.: 88, SU.51/128+ line 13.

48 Finkel 1998: 79–80, HS 1555+1587 rev. 16.

49 Finkel 1998: 79–80, HS 1555+1587 rev.17.

50 See in Finkel 1998:87–89, SU.51/128+ line 13. The part of the ox afflicted by the illness was the horn (gu$_4$ si-bi ba-ni-in-dab / *al-pu ina qar-ni -šú iṣ-bat*), whereas the sheep is always described as afflicted by the hoof, see Finkel 1998: 87–89, SU.51/128+ line 14.

51 Finkel 1998: 79–80, HS 1555+1587 rev. 14–17.

In incantation texts, it is indicated that the Samana-demon was highly contagious and prone to attacking animals that shared an enclosed space.[52] This was likely due to the close proximity and contact with excrements, a phenomenon discussed in Section 1 above.

To better understand the symptoms related to this disease, more clues can be found in the medical technical literature regarding humans, particularly in the diagnostic-prognostic series *Sakikkû*:

> DIŠ GIG GAR-*šú* SA$_5$ *e-em* MÚ-*iḫ* *u* G[IN-*a*]*k* *sa-ma-nu* [MU.NI]
> DIŠ GIG GAR-*šú* SA$_5$ LÚ KÚM.KÚM-*im u i-t*[*a-na*]*r*$^?$-*ru*$^?$ *sa-ma-nu* [MU.NI]
> DIŠ GIG GAR-*šú* *da-an* TAB ⸢x-*ma*⸣ *ina* IGI-*ka la i-na-aš* MÚD ŠUB KI.MIN *sa-ma-nu* MU.NI[53]
> If the disease, its appearance is red, hot, swollen and ⸢it flows⸣, [its name] is *samānu*.
> If the disease its appearance is red and the patient becomes feverish and repeatedly vomits, [its name] is *samānu*.
> If the disease its appearance is hard, it burns [. . .] and does not respond to the treatment, it bleeds; *ditto* its name is *samānu*.

The quoted lines provide significant information about the *samānu*-disease. Thus, it was characterized by redness, swelling, pus discharge, and fever, as confirmed by medical prescriptions for its treatment.[54]

Nevertheless, its identification in modern medical science is still uncertain. The etymology of the term has been linked to the word *sāmu* 'red', but as observed by J. V. Kinnier Wilson,[55] the red color was not the only one associated with this illness. Several identifications of *samānu* with modern biomedical equivalents have been proposed by researchers in past decades.[56] The Chicago Assyrian Dictionary defines *samānu* as an "ergot-like blight" that could affect humans, animals, and even barley.[57] J. V. Kinnier Wilson identified the *samānu*-disease with *mycetoma*, a fungal infection of the skin, which could affect feet, hands, and head.[58] Meanwhile, J. A. Scurlock and B. R. Andersen only described it as a soft tissue infection.[59] Finally, S. Beck recently[60] underlines that the symptomatic picture could correspond to various pathologies, although she considered *cutaneous leishmaniasis*, *pyodermas* such as *impetigo contagiosa* or furuncles, to be among the most probable identifications.[61]

According to Mesopotamian therapeutic literature, the symptoms associated with the *samānu*-disease suggest a contagious soft tissue infection characterized by redness, swelling, and pus discharge, as far as the observation of this disease in humans is concerned. Incantations, however, provide information about the presence of *samānu* in animals. It appears that oxen and sheep were most commonly affected, likely due to their confinement in small spaces. However, texts lack information on the symptoms observed in animals aside from the mention of anatomical parts that may be affected by *samānu*, such as the ox's palate, the sheep's hoof, the donkey's ear, and the stag's horn.

3 The Asakku-Demon

Asakku seems to be one of the most feared demons reported in incantation texts. It was described as a carrier of death and destruction, and a plague that strikes both humans and livestock. In the incantation series Udug-ḫul, Asakku appears as an evil demon (often alongside Namtar and Samana)[62] as well as a disease,[63] described as "disease

52 Finkel 1998: 82–83, A 7885 rev. 18 (gu$_4$ tùr-ra udu amaš-a im-mi-íb-kéš-a-ke$_4$-eš).
53 Heeßel 2000: 354, *Sakikkû* 33 lines 23–25
54 For redness, see BAM 409 obv. 11' (other colors such as black, yellow, and white are mentioned here), BAM 494 col. i 35', AMC line 61. For discharge of pus, see BAM 409 obv. 16' and AMC line 61.
55 Kinnier Wilson 1994: 111.
56 For a more comprehensive description of the history of research regarding the *samānu*-disease, see Scurlock and Andersen 2005: 692 n. 176.
57 CAD S: 112.
58 Kinnier Wilson 1994.
59 Surlock and Andersen 2005: 62.
60 Beck 2015.
61 Beck 2015: 38–46.
62 Bácskay 2013: 4.
63 á-sàg gig-ga/*asakku marṣu* (see e.g. UH III 128, VI 53, VII 40, XIII–XV 12, XVI 171). For further discussion of Asakku as a disease, see Böck 2014: 34–38 and Bácskay 2013.

of the eye"[64] and "illness not improving".[65] Additionally, as posited by M. Stol, the Asakku demon was also regarded as the cause of some terminal illnesses affecting women, particularly those associated with muscle pain.[66]

Yet Asakku is known first and foremost as the main antagonist of the Sumerian epic Lugal-e, in which this demon, as the carrier of chaos and destruction, fights the god Ninurta. In the poem, several references imply that Asakku was considered a disease, a plague and epidemic, and it is described as "a pustule whose suppuration is painful"[67] and a "rash that is not pleasant (to look at) when it comes out of the nose".[68]

Besides being the name of a disease and a demon, Asakku was also associated with violating a taboo.[69] The syntagm *asakka akālu* meaning "eating the *asakku*"[70] probably referred to the action of breaking an oath, and such a violation could be punished with terrible illness, perhaps personified by the demon Asakku. Despite the appearance of the Asakku-demon and *asakku*-disease in incantation texts, no clear symptomatology can be associated with the demon, and neither the demon nor the disease appear in medical texts or recipes for pharmacological treatments.

Still, the statement "death by Asakku" is widely attested outside the incantation texts and it was recognized as one of the principal causes of death of livestock in the administrative texts of the Ur III period.[71] In this documentation, death by *asakku* is described as RI.RI.GA[72] Á.SÀG or BA.UG$_7$ Á.SÀG.[73] However, these texts do not provide any practical information about the nature of the *asakku* disease or what was associated with death by Asakku. In the text DAS 50[74] as many as 225 sheep dead on account of *asakku* are reported.[75] However, only 184 dead sheep are specifically declared RI.RI.GA Á.SÀG in the text,[76] whereas the others are listed as dead (RI.RI.GA) without a specific cause. Consequently, it is reasonable to assume that no relevant differences were made between the sheep died by *asakku* and the others that simply died in the final tally. It is possible that the reason for the death of cattle or flocks was not considered significant enough to be recorded on the tablet. The explanation of death by *asakku* may have been used to justify losses due to a generic disease or as an act of the gods.

The reason why these deaths of livestock were reported as "death by Asakku" could be explained by the necessity of the farmer to justify the deaths of animals without blaming the caretaker, and as a reason for having the animal refunded.[77]

According to this study, the term "Asakku" refers to a demon, an illness, the violation of a taboo, and one of the main causes of death for livestock during the Ur III period. Although a wide range of symptoms is associated with this entity, it never appears in the actual therapeutic documentation and thus cannot be linked to any specific pathological condition.

4 Conclusion

This study examines the issue of zoonotic diseases in Mesopotamia, with a focus on case studies of two demons related to infectious diseases that attack both humans and animals: Samana and Asakku.

---

64 igi gig á-sàg sa-ma-ná (UH VI 57). For translation see Geller 2016: 230.

65 á-sàg gig-ga tu-ra nu-du$_{10}$-ga (see e.g. UH II 66, III 141, VI 61, XVI 171', XIII–XV 224'). For translation, see Geller 2016: 82, 120, 231, 532, 489.

66 Stol 2016: 445.

67 Seminara 2001: 116–117, Lugal-e line 268 (ù-bu-bu-ul è-a-bi nu-du$_{10}$-ga/ *bu-bu-ʾ-tú šá a-ṣu-šu la ṭa-a-bu*).

68 Seminara 2001: 117, Lugal-e line 269 (*ṣe-en-ni-tu$_4$ šá ina ap-pi a-ṣu-šu la dam-qu*).

69 Geller 2018: 293 n. 7.

70 CAD A 2: 327 "to infringe on a taboo". For a discussion of this topic, see Charpin 1997.

71 For a discussion of animals' death attributed to Asakku, see Heimpel 1995: 100–103.

72 RI.RI.GA = *miqittu* "epidemic, death among animals, dead animals", see CAD M/2: 100–102.

73 For attestations of RI.RI.GA Á.SÀG or BA.UG$_7$ Á.SÀG, see BDTNS 047317 = OIP 121 603 rev. i 7; BDTNS 058902 = BPOA 1 no. 1198 obv. i 3; BDTNS 021275 = ITT 4 no. 7805 obv. i 2; BDTNS 057973 = Nisaba 6 no. 13 obv. i 8, obv. ii 16,35, obv. iv 9,37, obv. v 20 and 34, rev. i 30, rev. ii 4; BDTNS 057986 = Nisaba 6 no. 31 obv. iii 23, rev. i 10; BDTNS 013222 = PDT 1 no. 515 rev. iii 15; BDTNS 031724 = TCTI 1 no. 740 obv. ii 2, obv. iv 14 and 20, obv. v 2 and 7, rev. i 19, rev. iii 20; BDTNS 031812 = TCTI 1 no. 897 obv. v 26, rev. i 16 and 26, rev. ii 2.

74 BDTNS 028419.

75 DAS 50 rev. v 21–22.

76 DAS 50 obv. ii 30–31, obv. iii 22–23 and 27–28, obv. v 8–9 and 16–17, obv. vi 31 and 35–36.

77 Heimpel 1995: 102–103.

Section 1 addressed the question of whether there was a concept of zoonosis in Mesopotamia.

Analysis of epistolary documentation, legal codes, and therapeutic literature, including incantations and rituals, showed that Mesopotamian healers were aware of the risk of contagion by proximity or contact, both for humans and for animals confined in pens and in contact with their excrement. Additionally, examination of letters and lexical lists revealed that the names of diseases known from therapeutic documentation concerning humans were the same as those associated with animals. However, there is a significant gap in the available documentation due to the absence of descriptions of symptoms observed in animals for these diseases. The acknowledgement of contagion through contact or proximity, and the fact that the agents considered responsible for the pathological condition were the same for humans and animals, leads us to hypothesize that there was indeed an awareness of the risks of zoonosis, according to the definition given at the beginning of Section 1: "infections or diseases that can be transmitted directly or indirectly between animals and humans".

Sections 2 and 3 analyzed the cases of two demons, Samana and Asakku, related to infectious diseases that affect both humans and animals. The Samana-demon was believed to cause a contagious disease called *samānu* afflicting both people and livestock. In therapeutic texts pertaining to humans, it is described as causing red wounds, high temperature, and discharge of blood or pus. Incantations and lexical lists provide more information about Samana as a demon attacking animals, especially oxen and sheep that were in close contact in pens. The physical symptoms of the disease were mostly located around the horns and hooves of animals. However, it is difficult to determine if *samānu*, as described in both humans and animals, is the same disease from a modern biomedical perspective due to the lack of symptom description in the animal kingdom. Additionally, the symptomatology associated with *samānu* in therapeutic literature concerning humans can be attributed to several modern diseases, making its identification problematic. In the Mesopotamian perspective, it is possible that the disease was considered the same for both humans and animals. This may have been due to the red color of its symptoms and its infectious nature.

In contrast, the Asakku-demon remains more enigmatic. The broad but generic symptomatology associated with this demon in incantation texts and the lack of references to Asakku in the medical literature have led to the assumption that the term did not refer to a specific disease. The creature may have been viewed as a general disruptive force, likely associated with epidemics or plagues, affecting both humans and animals. The Asakku-demon in the Lugal-e epic is often portrayed as a harbinger of chaos, destruction, and disease. Similarly, in Ur III period administrative texts, it was linked to the death of livestock. However, these texts do not provide any practical information about the nature of the *asakku* disease, nor do they distinguish between sheep that died from *asakku* and those that died from other causes. Therefore, it is possible that the term "death by Asakku", specifically RI.RI.GA Á.SÀG or BA.UG$_7$ Á.SÀG, was utilized to explain losses caused by general diseases or natural disasters.

In conclusion, this study has shown that the ancient Mesopotamians had a notion of infectious diseases that affected both humans and animals. Although it is difficult to identify such diseases with modern biomedical equivalents, the concept of zoonotic diseases may also have existed in Mesopotamia.

Bibliography

Arbøll 2018 = T. P. Arbøll, 'Tracing Mesopotamian Medical Knowledge: A Study of *maškadu-* and Related Illnesses', in: *Sources of Evil. Studies in Mesopotamian Exorcistic Lore*, ed. G. van Buylaere, M. Luukko, D. Schwemer and A. Mertens-Wagschal, Ancient Magic and Divination 15 (Leiden and Boston: Brill), 261–284

Arbøll 2021b = T. P. Arbøll, 'Were People in Ancient Mesopotamia Aware of Zoonoses?', in: *Eskiçağda Salgın ve Hstalıklar*, ed. Ö. S. Gavaz and G. M. Şahin (Istanbul: Yayına Hazıirlayanlar), 23–50

Arbøll 2024 = T T. P. Arbøll, 'Revisiting Epidemics in Cuneiform Sources: Ancient Attestations, Approaches, and Innovations', in: *Plague in Antiquity*, ed. L. Hitchcock, A. Jamieson, and C. Tully, Ancient Near Eastern Studies Supplement Series (Leuven, Paris, and Walpole: Peeters), 13–33

Bácskay 2013 = A. Bácskay, 'Asakkû: Demons and Illness in Ancient Mesopotamia', in: *Studies on Magic and Divination in the Biblical World*, ed. H. Jacobus, A. Gudme and P. Guillaume, Biblical Intersections 11 (New Jersey: Gorgias Press), 1–9

Biggs 1991 = R. D. Biggs, 'Ergotism and Other Mycotoxicoses in Ancient Mesopotamia?', *Aula Orientalis* 9, 15–21

Beck 2015 = S. Beck, 'Sāmānu as a Human Disease', *Journal des Médecines Cunéiformes* 26, 33–46

Birot 1993 = M. Birot, *Correspondance des gouverneurs de Qaṭṭunân*, Archives royales de Mari 27 (Paris: Librairie orientaliste Paul Geuthner)

Böck 2014 = B. Böck, *The Healing Goddess Gula: Towards an Understanding of Ancient Babylonian Medicine*, Culture and History of the Ancient Near East 67 (Leiden and Boston: Bsrill)

Charpin 1997 = D. Charpin, 'Manger un serment', in: *Jurer et maudire: pratiques politiques et usages juridiques du serment dans le Proche-Orient ancien*, ed. S. Lafont, Méditerranées 10–11 (Paris: L'Harmattan), 85–96

Dossin 1978 = G. Dossin, *Correspondance féminine*, Archives royales de Mari 10 (Paris: Librairie orientaliste Paul Geuthner)

Durand 1988 = J. M. Durand, *Archives épistolaires de Mari I/1*, Archives royales de Mari 26/1 (Paris: Librairie orientaliste Paul Geuthner)

Durand 2000 = J. M. Durand, *Les Documents épistolaires du palais de Mari III*, Littératures Anciennes du Proche-Orient 18 (Paris: Les Éditions du Cerf)

Feder 2016 = Y. Feder, 'Defilement, Disgust, and Disease, The Experiential Basis of Hittite and Akkadian Terms for Impurity', *Journal of the American Oriental Society* 136/1, 99–116

Feder 2022= Y. Feder, *Purity and Pollution in the Hebrew Bible*: *From Embodied Experience to Moral Metaphor* (Cambridge: Cambridge University Press)

Finkel 1998 = I. L. Finkel, 'A Study in Scarlet: Incantations against Samana', in: *Festschrift für Rykle Borger zu seinem 65. Geburtstag am 24. Mai 1994 - tikip santakki mala bašmu*, ed. S.M. Maul, Cuneiform Monographs 10 (Groningen: Styx Publications), 71–106

Frevel and Nihan 2013 = C. Frevel and C. Nihan, *Purity and the Forming of Religious Traditions in the Ancient Mediterranean World and Ancient Judaism*, Dynamics in the History of Religions 3 (Leiden and Boston: Brill)

Geller 2016 = M. J. Geller, *Healing Magic and Evil Demons* (Boston and Berlin: De Gruyter)

Geller 2018 = M. J. Geller, 'The Exorcist's Manual (KAR 44)', in: *Assyrian and Babylonian Scholarly Texts and Catalogues*, ed. U. Steinert, BAM 9 (Boston and Berlin: De Gruyter), 292–312

Guichard and Marti 2013 = M. Guichard and L. Marti, 'Purity in Ancient Mesopotamia. The Paleo-Babylonian and Neo-Assyrian periods', in: *Purity and the Forming of Religious Traditions in the Ancient Mediterranean World and Ancient Judaism*, ed. C. Frevel and C. Nihan, Dynamics in the History of Religions 3 (Leiden and Boston: Brill), 47–114.

Heimpel 1995 = W. Heimpel, 'Plow animal inspection records from Ur III Girsu and Umma', *Bulletin on Sumerian Aqriculture* 8/2, 71–171

Heimpel 1996 = W. Heimpel, 'hâšum to choke', *NABU* 1996/2, 40–41

Heeßel 2000 = N. P. Heeßel, *Babylonisch-assyrisch Diagnostik*, Alter Orient und Altes Testament 43 (Münster: Ugarit-Verlag)

Heeßel 2004 = N. P. Heeßel, 'Reading and Interpreting Medical Cuneiform Texts – Methods and Problems', *Journal des Médecines Cunéiformes* 3, 2–9.

Heeßel 2007 = N. P. Heeßel, 'The Hands of the Gods: Disease Names, and Divine Anger', in: *Disease in Babylonia*, eds. I. L. Finkel and M. J. Geller, Cuneiform Monographs 36 (Leiden and Boston: Brill), 120–130

Hoffner 1997 = H. A. Hoffner, *The Laws of the Hittites, A Critical Edition* (Leiden, New York, and Köln: Brill)

Kämmerer 1995 = T. R. Kämmerer, 'Die erste Pockendiagnose stammt aus Babylonien', *Ugarit-Forschungen* 27, 129–168

Kinnier Wilson 1994 = J. V. Kinnier Wilson, 'The Sāmānu Disease in Babylonian Medicine', *Journal of Near Eastern Studies* 53/2, 111–115

Nutton 2000 = V. Nutton, 'Did the Greeks have a Word for It? Contagion and Contagion Theory in Classical Antiquity', in: *Contagion: Perspectives from Pre-Modern Societies*, eds. L. Conrad and D. Wujastyk (Abingdon and New York: Routledge), 136–162

Oppenheim and Hartman 1945 = L. Oppenheim and L. F. Hartman, 'The Domestic Animals of Ancient Mesopotamia According to the XIII Tablet of the Series HAR.ra = *hubullû*', *Journal of Near Eastern Studies* 4/3, 152–177

Reiner 1958 = E. Reiner, *Šurpu, A Collection of Sumerian and Akkadian Incantations*, Archiv für Orientforschung Beiheft 11 (Osnabrück: Biblio Verlag)

Scurlock and Andersen 2005 = J.-A. Scurlock and B. R. Andersen, *Diagnoses in Assyrian and Babylonian Medicine. Ancient Sources, Translations, and Modern Medical Analyses* (Urbana and Chicago: University of Illinois Press)

Scurlock 2014 = J.-A. Scurlock, *Sourcebook for Ancient Mesopotamian Medicine*, Writings From the Ancient World 36 (Atlanta: SBL Press)

Seminara 2001 = S. Seminara, *La versione accadica del Lugal-e: La tecnica babilonese della traduzione dal sumerico e le sue 'regole'*, Materiali per il Vocabolario Sumerico 8 (Rome: Università degli Studi di Roma "La Sapeinza")

Steinert 2018 = U. Steinert, 'The Aššur Medical Catalogue', in: *Assyrian and Babylonian Scholarly Texts and Catalogues*, ed. U. Steinert, Die babylonisch-assyrische Medizin in Texten und Untersuchungen 9 (Boston and Berlin: De Gruyter), 203–291

Stadhouders 2012 = H. Stadhouders, 'The Pharmacopoeial Handbook Šammu šikinšu, A Translation', *Journal des Médecines Cunéiformes* 19, 1–21

Stol 2006–08 = M. Stol, 'Samana', in: *Reallexikon der Assyriologie und Vorderasiatischen Archäologie. Band 11. Prinz – Samug*, ed. M. P. Streck (Berlin: De Gruyter), 609–611

Stol 2016 = M. Stol, *Women in the Ancient Near East* (Boston and Berlin: De Gruyter)

Stol 2017 = M. Stol, 'Review of T. Abusch and D. Schwemer, Corpus of Mesopotamian Anti-Witchcraft Rituals. Volume 2 (Ancient Magic and Divination, 8/2)', *Bibliotheca Orientalis* 74/3–4, 371–379

Wasserman 2012 = N. Wasserman, 'Maškadum and other zoonotic diseases in medical and literary Akkadian sources', *Bibliotheca Orientalis* 69/5, 426–436

Yuhong 2001 = W. Yuhong, 'Rabies and Rabid Dogs in Sumerian and Akkadian Literature', *Journal of the American Oriental Society* 121/1, 32–43

2 Epidemic Outbreaks

Annie Attia

The Epidemics: How Were They Experienced in Day-to-Day Life in Mesopotamia?

Epidemics are calamities that have existed since the dawn of time, or at least since humankind gathered in larger or smaller groups. Mesopotamia, “the Cradle of Civilisation”, experienced and recorded many epidemics. In addition to technical medical texts, other documentation, such as letters, give an insight into how the ancients understood and experienced these episodes. Such tragedies spread throughout society and were the subject of letters allowing us to enter homes and share in this catastrophe. More generally, we can use other more sophisticated texts such as prayers or more common texts such as almanacs to understand how the ancients suffered from these epidemics on a day-to-day basis.

1 What is an Epidemic?

When browsing the internet, the definitions of epidemics are not unified. One can find a definition such as that of a French reference dictionary, the Robert, which associates propagation and infectious disease: “Apparition et propagation d’une maladie infectieuse contagieuse qui frappe en même temps et en un même endroit un grand nombre de personnes, d’animaux (épizootie) ou de plantes (épiphytie)”.[1] Or in the Concise Medical Dictionary: “A sudden outbreak of infectious disease that spreads rapidly through the population, affecting a large proportion of people”.[2] In contrast, there is no longer any mention of infectious disease on Merriam-Webster’s website: “an outbreak of disease that spreads quickly and affects many individuals at the same time”.[3] A clarification is added: “affecting many persons at the same time, and spreading from person to person in a locality where the disease is not permanently prevalent”.[4] In the Oxford handbook of Public Health Practice Sarah O’ Brien explains that: “The meaning of the term epidemic is broad. It encompasses both communicable diseases, e.g. meningitis, and non-communicable diseases, e.g. obesity . . . The numbers of cases, geographic extent, and time period need to be specified to be able to describe an epidemic” (O’Brien 2013: 166).

In the letters found in Mesopotamia, an epidemic is perceived as a disease provoking numerous simultaneous, rapid, and inexorable deaths. It is a deadly disease that spreads rapidly through populated areas. It was called *mūtānu*, which I translate as “the Deadly bringer”.[5] Interestingly and meaningfully, in Sumerian, it is rendered by úš.meš, nam. úš.meš, many deaths or much mortality.

2 The Patients: Who was Concerned? Who was Affected?

The ancient epidemics could strike everybody regardless of gender, age, social class, or rank. What was considered impressive was the significant number of deaths in a short time. In Mari, several letters illustrate the spread of epidemics among the population: “The household of your servant Bahlu-gayim has been wiped out in an epidemic (*ina ukulti ilim*

1 <https://dictionnaire.lerobert.com/definition/epidemie> (accessed 25/12/2021).
2 <https://oxfordmedicine.com/view/10.1093/med/9780199586301.001.0001/med-9780199586301-chapter-17> (accessed 25/12/2021).
3 <https://www.merriam-webster.com/dictionary/epidemic> (accessed 25/12/2021).
4 <https://www.merriam-webster.com/words-at-play/epidemic-vs-pandemic-difference> (accessed 25/12/2021).
5 This translation fits the context, though some might consider it unconventional; another had been proposed by Jean Bottéro (1978: 135), the “male-mort”. This French ancient term for a tragic and merciless death was used to designate plague. Unfortunately, I have not found an English equivalent for this perfectly adapted expression for the notion of *mūtānu*. In general, the term is regarded as a plural of the word for death and often translated as “cases of death, epidemic, pestilence, plague”.

Annie Attia, UMR 7192, Paris

 | https://doi.org/10.1515/9783112238622-004

'devouring-by-a-god'); all his children died. No one remains to be responsible for the household".[6] Deaths due to the spread of an epidemic were regularly recorded: "About the 'devouring by a god' (. . .), in Tuttul there is disease, but death is rare. In Dunnum, below Lasqum, there is a *heap of dead.* Within two days, about 20 people died",[7] and in another letter: "In one day, 10 men and 5 children died".[8]

In the Neo-Assyrian archives from Nineveh we find reports about sun eclipses with deadly prediction, such as: "there will be deaths within one day".[9] And in an *Astronomical Diary* from Babylon, Parthian period BM 32884 (-93A) obv. 11: "[. . .] That month, there were many sick (gig.meš) and dead (úš.meš) in the land".[10]

The soldiers, men in the prime of their lives, were not spared. In Mari, due to the concentration of men in the army, the plague was widespread, as reported in a letter: "I gave 20 small-boats on which to embark the sick (soldiers). Then, I realized how many sick people there were among them. Those small-boats were not enough for them. So I gave them 2 large-boats for their need".[11]

In the palace, the epidemic caused suffering as well, and in the harem of King Zimri-Lim, letters explain the actions undertaken to prevent the spread of diseases and protect women from being contaminated. One letter concerns a woman called Summudum:

> "About Summudum, the subject of your letter, because of this woman's illness, many women will be sick with this *simmum*-ailment. This woman must live in a separate room. Let no one visit her! But if, as I fear, there is no separate room, as long as the omens (*têrētum*: doctor's report or extispicy) concerning Summudum are not favourable, why bother with this woman? Whether she dies or lives, there are women who will be sick (*imarraṣā*) with this *simmum*-ailment. Therefore, let this woman die, alone!"[12]

In a later episode, recorded in the Amarna archives, an epidemic enters the Pharaoh's harem and kills his wives. Letters report the death of two foreign wives of Pharaoh Amenhotep III, father of Akhenaten. Specifically, a daughter of Burna-buriash, king of Babylon[13] and Kelukhepa, a Mitanian princess,[14] died, and Akhenaten requested their respective fathers to replace them. Does this reflect reality or is it a lie to cover up ill-treatment? The balance is in favour of an epidemic because, at the same time, we feel the pain of a Cypriot king when he writes to the Pharaoh: "My brother, do not worry if your messenger has stayed three years in my country, for the Hand of Nergal (šu-ti ^{d}maš.maš) is in my country, and in my own house I had a young wife who now, my brother, is dead".[15] In this period, Murshili II, a Hittite sovereign, also explains that Egyptian prisoners brought back to Hatti were at a major epidemic's origin ("Second Prayer" see further on).

Animals, too, could be afflicted during epidemics. Cattle, sheep, horses and farmyard animals could die in large numbers, which was recognised as the effects of epidemic diseases. There are examples of predictions of abnormally high mortality in flocks, which is indirect evidence of the occurrence of epidemic diseases. Farmers or herders were able to identify these particular diseases. One example of plague prediction is KUB 4 no. 63 (col. iii 16): "If there is a solar eclipse in Arahsamna there will be an epidemic among the cattle, an outbreak of the *samānu*-illness" (*miqitti* (ri.ri.ga) *būl Šakkan ukulti samānim,* Leibovici 1956: 11–21).

In Mari, a plague broke out killing men and animals: "The god undertook in Kulhitum to devour oxen and the population (*ilum ana akāl alpī u awīlūtim qātam iškun*); during the day, 2 to 3 men died".[16] A gloomy story of diseased and

6 ARM 5 no. 87 obv. 5–13, translation follows FMA: 334. For transcription, French translation, and bibliography of this Mari text see the Archibab website <https://www.archibab.fr/T8418> (accessed 27/03/2020).

7 ARM 26/1 no. 259 obv. 5–14, see <https://www.archibab.fr/T7415> (accessed 09/04/2022).

8 ARM 26/1 no. 260 obv. 7–8, see <https://www.archibab.fr/T7416> (accessed 01/03/2022).

9 SAA 8 no. 384 r 4. For transcription, English translation and bibliography of the State Archive of Assyria, see the ORACC website for SAAo <http://oracc.org/saao/P237900/> (accessed 27/03/2020).

10 Sachs and Hunger 1996: 428; see *Astronomical Diaries Digital on ORACC* <https://oracc.museum.upenn.edu/adsd/adart3/akk?xis=akk.r0003ed&ref=X300931.12> (accessed 29/07/2022).

11 ARM 26/1 no. 274, see <https://www.archibab.fr/T7430> (accessed 10/04/2022).

12 LAPO 18: 346; ARM 10 no. 130, see <https://www.archibab.fr/T8686> (accessed 10/04/2022).

13 EA 10, see Moran 1992, 19–20 (translation). Transcription and bibliography of the Amarna letters can be found on the ORACC website <http://oracc.museum.upenn.edu/contrib/amarna/corpus> (accessed 10/04/2022).

14 EA 19, see Moran 1992, 43–46 (translation).

15 EA 35, see Moran 1992, 107–109 (translation).

16 ARM 3 no. 61 rev. 9–13, see <https://www.archibab.fr/T8091> (accessed 13/01/2022).

quarantined sheep also occurs at Tell Leilan in Syria, at the end of the second millennia BCE. A letter shows the difficulties faced by a shepherd with his flock in finding a place to graze after an epidemic disease prevented him from moving his sheep:

> "Previously I wrote to you about my sheep, and you said: "Place your sheep in Ahanda, let (them) go there". This, my elder brother told me. The sheep (were ready) to be led to Ahanda, but the god struck my sheep (*ilum ilput*)[17], and until I appeased the god (*adi ilam ušallimu*), I kept (them) back, but (then) the sheep of Nilibšinnum were placed in Ahanda. Afterward, when I had appeased the god, Yaqbiya, the chief shepherd, indicated the town of Kuzāya for the sheep; the sheep were placed in Kuzāya, but the *sugāgum* of Kuzāya chased my sheep away. Now will my elder brother please send his retainer with my retainer, so they will not chase away my sheep in Kuzāya."[18]

In the shepherd's letter the god responsible for the plague is not named. In other contexts the gods are mentioned specifically. In a letter to the king Esarhaddon, an astrologer explains various predictions as follows: "If the day is gloomy and rides the north wind: devouring by Nergal, the cattle will diminish".[19] The plague and war god Erra was responsible for epizootics – epidemics in animals – in a royal inscription of Ashurbanipal: "Like the carnage of the god Erra, the bodies (and) corpses of oxen and s[*heep and goats*] were heaped up [*in the stepp*]e and open country".[20]

3 How Did the People Affected by Epidemics React? What Questions Did They Ask?

One of the first questions a person suffering from an illness asks is "why is this happening? Why is it happening to me?" The letters help us understand today how the ancients tried to answer such questions. The names given to the epidemics constitute the first step in answering the first question. As previously discussed, an epidemic was generally called *mūtānu*, the Deadly bringer. In Mari the epidemic is also called "*qāt ilim* Hand of the god", and it could touch or strike (*lapātu*) or be placed, settled (*šaknu*). The god involved is not called by name and remains anonymous.

Elsewhere, Nergal, the god of death, could be held responsible for these calamities, but also Erra, as mentioned above. But, other gods were also involved. In a letter dated to the same period as those from Mari, originating in Umma in southern Babylonia, an inquiry is made to identify the god responsible for the epidemic. Nergal was ruled out as the cause of the epidemic, which was attributed to another god, Asari (i.e., Marduk):

> Behold, there is a deadly epidemic (*mu-ta-a-nu*) in the city. It is not an epidemic (*mu-ta-a-nu*) of the god Nergal. It is an epidemic (*mu-ta-a-nu*) of Asari (Marduk) [. . .]. Let the herald cry out: 'Hold *gatherings*[21] in a closed place for Asari and make the god favourable to you!' May the god be calmed during the *gatherings*![22]

In Larsa, a prayer-letter is addressed to the sun god in order to stop an epidemic. The king begs the god Shamash to end an epidemic that has plagued his city for seven years.[23] The king describes a city with its wide streets, now empty and silent. He complains that his young people are affected while enemy troops are unharmed. In this way, he makes the same association between war and epidemic that occurs in other places and at other times. The king denies having acted wrongly. Unlike his enemies, he has been respectful of the deities and has followed carefully religious regulations. Accordingly, he does not understand why Shamash, the god of justice, strikes him.[24] This revolt against divine arbitrariness is most interesting on the part of a king and should be compared with the resignation of Šubši-mešrê-Šakkan in *Ludlul bēl nēmeqi*.[25]

---

17 The verb *lapātu* (CAD L: 82–94) means "to touch", and by extension, *lipit ilim* is employed in the context of epidemic (CAD L: 201–202).

18 Eidem 2011: 156–157 text 85.

19 SAA 10 no. 79, see <http://oracc.org/saao/P334276/> (accessed 10/04/2022).

20 RINAPo Ashurbanipal 186 line 30, see <http://oracc.org/rinap/Q007594/> (accessed 10/04/2022).

21 See Arbøll (2024: 17 n. 32) for the translation of *taphūrū*. Note that the word is a hapax legomenon.

22 AbB 2 no. 118, see <https://www.archibab.fr/ T16551> (accessed 10/04/2022).

23 "Appeal to Utu II", see Hallo 1976: 209–224.

24 About this epidemic, notice its reconstruction by Goodnick-Westenholz 1983: 223 n. 22 with bibliography.

25 For the acceptance or resignation of human beings when faced with the injustice of evil, which strikes good and bad alike, see Oshima and Anthonioz 2023. For a "medical" vision of the doomed fate of the *Ludlul* hero, see Attia 2018: 55–58.

In the late 2nd millennium BCE Amarna archive, as well as the Neo-Assyrian archives of Nineveh, epidemics are mainly the work of the god Nergal. Such plagues were one of the curses inflicted upon those who broke a treaty or opposed a royal decision, as exemplified in the following example from the Tell Tayinat version of Esarhaddon's succession treaty: "May Nergal, hero of the gods, extinguish your life with his merciless sword, and [s]end slaughter (*šaggaštu*) and pestilence (nam.úš^{meš}, *mūtānu*) among you".[26]

The god Erra was also linked to violent death, and he was implicated in the genesis of epidemics. The touch of this god could cause epidemic diseases in humans and animals, as shown in a literary text: "He who in his heart plots evil against the king – Erra will call him to account through plague (*šibṭi*) (and) slaughter (*šaggašti*)".[27] Further illustrating the point, a letter containing an astrological report states: "(If) in Nisannu an eclipse [. . .] in the evening watch: [. . .]; alternatively, Erra will devour (gu$_7$ = *ikkal*)".[28] Other gods may be involved in these ravaging diseases.

Therefore, the first answer to the initial question is that the gods were responsible for the appearance and spread of deadly diseases. But why did the gods send this evil death? In Mari, there is no clear answer. In the correspondence, there is no trace of a search for the failure that might have caused it, one is merely aware of the existence of the epidemic and endures it. The god responsible in Mari was depicted as a devourer, an ogre: "*aš-šum ú-ku-ul-ti* dingir-*lim*".[29] He would be a kind of merciless glutton who would feed on human flesh.[30]

In later omen series, the plague was still described as the devouring by a god. Nicla de Zorzi has pointed out in her article about the omen series *Šumma izbum*[31] that comparison with predatory animals like wolf or dogs led to predictions of plague, discord, and strife: "If a goat gives birth to a wolf the god will devour (*ilu ikkal* pestilence)"[32] or "If an ewe gives birth to a lion, and it has the head of a dog, Nergal will devour (*Nergal ikkal*)" (Leichty 1978: 78 tablet v: 54). Similarly, one finds the following omen in *Šumma ālu*: "If bitches bark in gates, devouring by Erra (*ukulti Erra*) will be all over the land" (Ālu 48 line 1, Freedman 2017: 66).

The metaphor of devouring is understandable in the context of carnivorous animals preying on humans.[33] Still, there are presumably some unfortunate human experiences behind this terrifying image. For example, several descriptions of cannibalism, as well as dogs and pigs feeding on corpses, are known from the Neo-Assyrian royal inscriptions.[34] Consequently, the metaphor of devouring may originate in actual experience when walking through plague ravaged streets. In this respect, the description given by Ashurbanipal is highly evocative (see n. 34). These horrible images could have been on everyone's mind, and must have made epidemics and supernatural forces seem threatening. One also wonders whether the "devouring gods"-epidemic was also hinting to a lack of sustenance that men owed to the deities, as cults were probably not well maintained in such times of crisis. It can also refer to a human failure to fulfil the duty of care owed to the divinity.

But in other contexts, the responsibility lies within human behaviour, such as transgression and wrong doing. It is implicit in the royal curses, that any breach of promise or loyalty was punishable by plague. The idea of divine punishment is found in several documents. One of the most impressive of these, however, is the plague prayers written by the Hittite king Mursili II (1321–1295 BCE).[35] After his father's (Suppiluliuma I) victorious battle against the Egyptian army, the prisoners brought back to Hatti were regarded as the cause of a terrible epidemic (see "Second prayer"). Surprisingly, the Hittite gods allowed this plague to spread. Their anger was apparently provoked by a crime committed by

26 SAA 2 no. 15 § 49 455 T vi 35, see <http://oracc.org/saao/P500551/> (accessed 10/04/2022).

27 SAA 3 no. 11 rev. 11, <http://oracc.org/saao/P336242/> (accessed 10/04/2022).

28 CTN 4 no. 29 obv.12–13, see <http://oracc.org/cams/gkab/P363444> (accessed 15/04/2022).

29 ARM 26/1 no. 259 See <https://www.archibab.fr/T7415> (accessed 09/04/2022).

30 See Durand 1988: 548–549 n. 29 on this point. His remark that the fact that verb *akālu* is used to express that the enemies are ravaging the country is particularly significant.

31 De Zorzi, 2011: 43–75.

32 Tablet xviii line 17'. Notice that De Zorzi 2011: 62 reads or restores *ikkal*.

33 See Esztári 2018: 32.

34 RINAPo Ashurbanipal 011: (iv 41b–45b) "At that time, (as for) the people of the land Akkad who had sided with Šamaš-šuma-ukīn (and) plotted evil (deeds), hunger took hold of them. They ate the flesh of their sons (and) their daughters on account of their hunger; they gnawed on (leather) straps." And iv 79–84"I brought out of Babylon, Cutha, (and) Sippar the bones of the people's corpses that the god Erra had cut down and those who had laid down (their) live(s) from famine (and) starvation, the remnants of meal(s) for dogs (and) pigs, which were obstructing the streets (and) filling the squares", see <http://oracc.org/rinap/Q003710/> (accessed 03/03/2021).

35 This epidemic and its consequences have given rise to several prayers describing its origin, evolution, and causes. Conventionally, these prayers are named by their respective numbers. See their transcriptions and translations in Beckman 2003:156–160.

Mursili's father during a conspiracy. Mursili, in the "First Prayer", blames his father's wrongdoing for this divine wrath.[36] In his "Third Prayer", the king implores and begs the gods to put an end to it while simultaneously emphasizing the length of the epidemic: "You have let the plague enter Hatti . . . so that Hatti has been hit hard by the plague . . . This is the twentieth year that people are dying in Hatti".[37]

With the epidemic hitting everyone equally, we can address the final question of "why me", and whether this ever arose? To my knowledge, it seems that this issue has left no trace. The epidemic appears to be a "general" punishment or the result of an evil predisposition, such as that announced by an eclipse, an evil sunrise, a malicious configuration in hepatoscopy, or other sinister omens. The wrongdoing of a ruler could provoke it, but this fault turned against his city or his whole country. However, everyone tried to protect themselves from this scourge with various devices which belong to the science of the exorcist and, accessorily, of the doctor, which I will not go into here.[38]

This observation naturally leads to another question that the Mesopotamians must have asked themselves: what can be done? And, effectively, what did they do?

By definition, for them, such diseases were beyond cure. Therefore, they tried, by all means available to them, to avoid being contaminated. As Durand (1988: 546) states concerning the Mari archives: "Nulle part, on ne voit les gens lutter sur place contre le mal par un moyen quelconque, fût-il religieux".[39]

In Mari, two main reactions are attested. The first was to flee the place of the epidemic, and the second to isolate the sick and not to have contact with them. Trying to appease the god who sent the plague was also believed to be helpful. Desperate to leave the towns where the epidemic was spreading, some people took refuge in safe, unharmed, and eventually uncrowded areas: "The people of Dunnum abandoned the city, escaping to Mt. Lasqum".[40] However, escape was forbidden for fear of spreading the disease, and people, especially the king, were warned against entering an infected area. For example, the diviner Ašqudum advised the king Zimri-Lim as follows:

> "God is striking in the upper district (*ilum ina halṣ[im el]îm u[l]appatma*) (. . .). My Lord must give orders that city-dwellers, once they are stricken (*laptū*), ought not to enter uninfected towns (*lā laptūtim*). The fear is that they will infect (*ulappatū*) the whole land. (. . .) My Lord must stop in Terqa and not proceed toward Saggaratum. The land (there) is infected (*lupputat*)."[41]

In later records, we find a similar apprehension about entering towns or territories where an epidemic is propagating. In the Amarna archives, in a letter sent from Byblos, the inhabitants of a contaminated city are prevented from entering a healthy city: "I will not permit men from Sumur to enter my city. There is a plague in Sumur".[42] It appears that this ban did not stop the epidemic from reaching Byblos. The denial of its existence by the city's king proves this: "As to his having said before the king, 'There is a plague (*mu-ta-ni*) in the lands.' (. . .) There is no plague (*mu-ta-na*) in the lands. All is healthy for a long time".[43]

When a sick person was discovered, confinement was organized to prevent the spreading of contamination. In Mari, the king, Zimri-Lim gives these instructions to his wife, Šibtu, about a certain Nanna, a harem woman (a servant):[44]

36 Singer 2021: 66–67: "En los textos se evidencia la búsqueda de una razón para explicar la peste que aflige al país. En la Primera Plegaria por la Peste, Mursili II expresa su culpa por el destino de Tudhaliya, el hijo menor del rey Tudhaliya, y el hermano menor y sucesor de Arnuwanda I, que fue asesinado junto con algunos de sus seguidores durante una conspiración dentro de la familia real."

37 See articles with pictures concerning this plague at <https://www.thecollector.com/the-plague-prayers-hittites/> and <https://www.dailysabah.com/arts/ancient-tablet-exhibit-to-tell-story-of-epidemics-in-anatolia/news> (accessed 12/01/2024).

38 See e.g. Maul 1999: 123–129.

39 "Nowhere do you see people fighting evil on the ground by any means, even religious ones."

40 ARM 26/1 no. 259 lines 15–18, see https://www.archibab.fr/T7415 (accessed 09/04/2022). Translation according to FMA: 333. Lasqum was a rocky place full of basalt stones. For this toponymal see Ziegler and Langlois 2016: 201–202; Stol 1979: 86; Groneberg 1980: 152.

41 ARM 26/1 no. 17 lines 20–30, see <https://www.archibab.fr/T7116> (accessed 09/03/2022).

42 EA 96, see Moran 1992: 170 (translation).

43 EA 362, see Moran 1992: 359–361 (translation).

44 The fact that this woman is a water fetcher is explained in Archibab concerning ARM 10 no. 129 n. 6–7 with reference to Ziegler (1999: 113), which can be consulted for details.

> "Since she is often at the palace, she connects many women through her. Now give strict orders: No one is to drink from the cup she uses; no one is to sit on the seat she takes; no one is to lie on the bed she uses, lest it infect the many women who are with her. This is a very contagious infection (*muštahhizu*)!"[45]

In another letter, Šibtu informs her husband of a severely ill woman in the harem. The prognosis is extremely unfavourable, and the risk of contamination is high, so the queen decides to isolate her:

> ". . . said to me: 'The woman, even if we touch her, will not live'. I asked her name. This woman is (a certain) Aštakka. For the time being, I have her living in the new buildings. She takes her beer and bread separately. No one is allowed to go near her bed or her seat'."[46]

It was feared that the disease would spread in the harem, which reminds us that densely populated places were known to be at risk. These letters demonstrate that these epidemics were transmitted by contact or sharing food. Even the objects touched by these women were considered dangerous. Through contact, or a violent or non-violent touch, the gods provoked the rise of epidemics. Accordingly, the ancients spoke of the hand of the god touching or striking the country (*lapātum*).

Letters, such as the ones quoted above, emphasize the desire for isolation, as people were well aware of the spread of certain diseases, particularly skin diseases as seen above.[47] The question is whether they had a notion of the contagiousness of an illness, some of the sickness somehow being transmitted by contact, or whether they feared contamination through the transmission of a transgression that made the individual impure. This sin could be responsible for the installation of a deadly disease. In my view, the most likely interpretation is that a stigma was passed on from one individual to another, and this had to be avoided. As Durand (1988: 546) explains: "Le contact qui est évité avec celui qui est 'touché' (*laptum*) par la 'Main-du-Dieu' vise non pas à se protéger contre une source de contagion purement physique, mais à se désolidariser de quelqu'un qui est moralement impur". It is equally probable, as Geller suggests (2010: 69), that they tried to bury the dead people as soon as possible in order to protect themselves from impure transmission.

The idea that disease can be transmitted by contact remained in later periods. This evoked for Walter Farber (2004: 117–132), in his article 'How to Marry a Disease', some useful thoughts on how diseases were supposed to be transferred. He noted that sorcerers made people eat or drink food that they had made harmful, by massages, or creating objects rendered evil. It explains why objects from the patients' daily lives were destroyed by fire in some major rituals, such as the *Šurpu*-burning ritual.[48]

The transmissibility of an epidemic, as well as its untreatable nature, had a detrimental effect on human relations by reducing social interaction, as evidenced by a prediction based on an abnormal birth: "If a malformed foetus his face is shaped like a wolf, there will be a severe deadly epidemic (*mūtānum dannūtum*) and people will no longer enter each other's homes (*ahum ana bīt ahim*)".[49] Even long-time friends or neighbours could develop feelings of enmity towards one another: "the god will devour (dingir gu_7), one street will be hostile to the other; one house will plunder the other".[50]

4 Economy

What emerges, in particular from the letters, is the economic impact of epidemics. As we have seen, regardless of age, sex, or social position, both the innocent and the guilty could be affected and die. Of course, the spectacular mortality of the epidemics was frightening, as no one was safe. But these plagues also affected the finances of citizens and sovereigns. The first impact consisted of a loss of staff, about which the administrators complain. It justifies why they counted the dead. In Mari, a letter from a certain Mašiya to his lord (Yasmah-Addu) elaborates: "Since the Hand of God which

45 LAPO 18: 345–6; ARM 10 no. 129, see <https://www.archibab.fr/T8685> (accessed 09/03/2022). Translation according to FMA: 331.

46 LAPO 18: 344 with collations and notes; ARM 10 no. 14, see <https://www.archibab.fr/T8684> (accessed 09/03/2022).

47 For *simmum* especially in Mari letters, see Durand 1988: 544, 551–552 and Attia and Buisson 2005: 42 n. a.

48 For the *Šurpu* ritual see Reiner 1958.

49 YOS 10 no. 56 col. iii 3–5 OB *Šumma izbu*, see Leichty (1970: 205).

50 *Šumma izbu* tablet 1: 82, see Leichty (1970: 39).

(was) on the country has calmed down, I had a tablet written on the deceased personnel, concerning the weavers, the agricultural workers, the . . . and the workshops".[51]

Similarly, a person named Sumu-hadu writes to his lord (Zimri-Lim) about the economic problems associated with an epidemic that is being propagated among the people: "Now, diseases are multiplying in the kingdom of Mari; many people are vomiting (*ṣabum hâšum mād*).[52] There is no house where there is no sick person. That which (constitutes) the grain of the Palace, for lack of people so far, has not been reaped".[53]

In later records, epidemics serve as a pretext for not satisfying official requests. Thus, the king of Cyprus explains to the pharaoh in a letter from Amarna that, because of a plague, his shipment of copper will be less substantial than expected:

> "I, herewith, have sent to you five hundred (talents or ingots) of copper. As my brother's greeting-gift, I have sent it to you. My brother, do not feel concern that the amount of copper is small. Behold the 'hand of Nergal' (or a local deity, šu-ti ᵈmaš.maš), my lord, is in my country. He has slain all the men of my country, and there is not a (single) copper-worker."[54]

The same tactic was used in Ṣumur (located in modern Syria), where the epidemic became the pretext not to send donkeys, as had otherwise been agreed:

> "Inasmuch as you say, 'I will not allow men of Ṣumur to enter [into] my city. An epidemic (*mu-ta-nu-mi*) is in Ṣumur.' It is an epidemic (*mu-ta-nu-ú*) with regard to men or *with regard to* donkeys? What is the epidemic (*mu-ta-nu*) with regard to donkeys [th]a[t] the donkeys *did not go* (into the city)? *Did they look for the king's donkeys? But no!* The king's possessions are lost."[55]

5 Inconsistences, Irrelevance, and Contradictions

In conclusion, I must admit that the "non-scientific" documentation, represented by the letters, also provides us with information that seems to contradict some statements made above. An epidemic has different names that appear to describe conditions with specific symptomatology rather than a disease characterised solely by its sudden and inevitable death.

In a letter (SAA 10 no. 296 obv. 11–12) the exorcist Nabu-naṣir informs the king of a performed ritual, and here, three illnesses related to an epidemic condition are quoted together: *di'u, mūtānu, šibṭu*. In teratological omens, the term *bibbu* also designates an epidemic.[56] *Masla'tu* could be an epidemic disease spreading in the army; its name derives from *salā'u*.[57]

For animals, *miqittu* could refer to an epidemic (or epizootic disease), but as this term can indicate other diseases and injuries, it should therefore be translated with caution (see Durand 1988: 548 n. 43)

Finally, treatments for incurable illness caused by an epidemic can be found in the scientific corpus, and maybe even in the letters as well. For example, Goodnick-Westenholz quotes a letter mentioning that no doctor is available, probably due to an epidemic or a highly contagious disease ravaging Babylonia.[58]

"Même pas peur" – Not even scared! To counter the notion that people are always afraid of an epidemic, we can point to the fact that it is only mentioned in passing in several documents. In the Assyrian Eponym Chronicle, three

51 ARM 26/1 no. 264 obv. 5–8, see <https://www.archibab.fr/T7420> (accessed 09/03/2022). Translated according to FMA: 334.

52 Jean-Marie Durand (2000: 118) commented on this word. The background was that of a fattened ox experiencing this problem. He derives the verb from *âšum* vomit (to be nauseous) rather than *hâšum*, meaning, to be in a mess.

53 ARM 33 no. 175 rev. 32–38, see <https://www.archibab.fr/T23847> (accessed 09/03/2022).

54 EA 35 obv. 10–14, see Moran 1992, 107–109 (translation).

55 EA 96 obv. 6–rev. 21, see Moran 1992, 170 (translation).

56 E.g. Leichty (1970: 201), YOS 10 no. 56 col. i 6–7: "There will be plague in the country" *bibbum ina mātim ibbašši*. Note also the late astrological text LBAT 1593 line 12', not quoted in CAD B.

57 Stol 2009: 46.

58 Goodnick-Westenholz 1983: 223 n. 22 quoted verbatim: "It seems possible that disease on an epidemic scale raged through Babylonia. Nādin-Ishtar writes to Ikūppīša to send a doctor to examine a case of *simmum* since there is no other doctor around (?) (Khalid Al-A'dami, 'Old Babylonian Letters from ed-Der,' *Sumer* 23 [1967]: 157). The description of Uruk as a dead city would be especially apt if it had been ravaged by disease. As pertaining to the health of Sumu-El might be seen the dedication of a dog by a gala-mah of Girsu for the life of Sumu-El to the

epidemic outbreaks were listed from 858 until 824 BCE (34 years). For 802 BC, the text states: "[Aššur-balti-ekurri governor of] Arrapḫa = to the Sea; plague"; in 765 BC: "Ninurta-mukīn-nišī governor of Ḫabrūri = to Ḫatarikka; plague"; and in 759 BC: "Pān-Aššur-lāmur governor of Arbail = rebellion in Gūzāna; plague".[59]

Furthermore, epidemic episodes are mentioned in almanacs, and in the names of eponymous years, but always in passing, such as the astronomical diary (AD -330A obv. 4'): "[. . .] during totality the west wind blew, during clearing the east wind. [. . .] fourth? . . .; during the eclipse, deaths (nam.úš.meš) and plague?(*šib-ṭu*) [occurred?] in [. . .]" Babylon, Hellenistic.[60]

In a letter from a governor to the king the experienced epidemic is a simple, relatively commonplace episode that allows them to use the event as a timeframe: "When there was an [ep]idemic (*mūtānu*) here, Ilu-bi'di, a cohort commander under my jurisdiction killed a horse. I made up for the horse in his stead and he promised: 'I'll give you the money'".[61]

The "les animaux malades de la peste", to quote a fable written by Jean de la Fontaine,[62] were not taboo for utilization and even for consumption. The report YOS 7 no. 96,[63] a "police" investigation from Uruk dated to the Persian period (Cambyses), concerns the cattle herds of the Eanna temple in Uruk. It mentions a *šibṭu*-epidemic that occurred there, resulting in the death of 21 animals. Not only did the herdsman not report this episode to the temple administrators, but he found buyers to the deceased cattle and sold the carcasses and hides. He defends himself by saying that he has not yet received money from the sale. According to him, this would justify that he has not referred the matter. Contrary to the above-mentioned texts, no taboo and no precaution is taken concerning these animals that died of the plague. In a recent article, Francis Joannès (2022) tried to determine the contagious disease that was decimating the herd. He explains that the carcasses were sold at a derisory price, and that buyers might have decided to ignore the illicit nature of the sale and the threat of taboo and contagion.

After these last quotes, I believe that what Leo Oppenheim wrote in "Mesopotamia, the portrait of a dead civilization" (1977: 24–25) is still relevant today, also for the present discussion: "The picture that any investigation based on such material can obtain consists of a number of spots of light. It is as if narrowly confined beam of light haphazardly illuminated this or that city between the Persian Gulf and the Mediterranean Sea at infrequent and irregular intervals during two millennia, leaving everything else in the darkness". There is a similar sense of frustration with the documentation discussed above, which is both impressive in its quality though fragmentary in its distribution. In his epilogue, Oppenheim (1977: 334) warns against the characteristics of this knowledge, comparable to Rorschach stains, the interpretation of which can end up reflecting only the reader's convictions.

6 To End on a Positive Note

Though we can rarely assess the modern epidemics behind outbreaks of ancient plagues, recent archaeogenetic studies challenge the desire to void identifying infectious causes of ancient epidemics. Already Singer (2017 and 2021) relied on tomb findings at Amarna showing that malaria was widespread and responsible for an increase in mortality and a weakening of the population. She mentions the discovery of indirect evidence of the bubonic plague in the population. The bacterium responsible for the Black Death was found in fossilised flies. As flies were the reservoir of the plague bacillus, this suggests that the pest could have been active at that period and was the cause of the great epidemic that affected the Levant and Turkey. A new study, published in Current Biology (Neumann et al. 2022), explains that "ancestors" of the bacteria responsible for the Black Death and dysentery existed in the third millennium BCE: "Here, we pres-

healing goddess Nin-isinna (see Durand, *RA* 71, pp. 32 ff.). The last piece of evidence might be cited from Kisurra letter 148 in which it is stated that Sumu-El is sick. The disease itself might possibly be described in the unknown word *ik-zu*; note the *mūti ik-zu* in l. 8."

59 On ORACC Textual Sources of the Assyrian Empire, <http://oracc.org/saao/Q007771/> (accessed 09/04/2022).

60 On ORACC Astronomical Diaries Digital, <https://oracc.museum.upenn.edu/adsd/corpus> (accessed 09/04/2022); see also Sachs and Hunger 1988: 176–177.

61 SAA 19 no. 171 obv. 14–rev. 5, see <http://oracc.org/saao/X190171/> (accessed 24/09/2022).

62 <https://gallica.bnf.fr/essentiels/fontaine/fables/animaux-malades-peste> (accessed 19/05/2022).

63 See Joannès 2022 and the following webpage <http://www.achemenet.com/fr/item/?/sources-textuelles/textes-par-regions/babylonie/uruk-larsa-ur/3631122> (accessed 12/01/2024).

ent genetic evidence for the presence of Yersinia pestis and Salmonella enterica, the causative agent of typhoid/enteric fever, from this period of transformation in Crete, detected at the cave site Hagios Charalambos". The authors acknowledge that despite some distance to Mesopotamia proper, current research tend to ignore the virulence and transmissibility of these bacteria. Accordingly, their detection is essential to keep in mind when dealing with ancient pathology, particularly with epidemics. And it is encouraging to think that science has not said its last word!

Bibliography

Al-A'dami 1967 = K. Al-A'dami, "Old Babylonian Letters from ed-Der", *Sumer* 23: 151–165 and pls.1–17

Arbøll 2024 = T. P. Arbøll, 'Revisiting Epidemics in Cuneiform Sources: Ancient Attestations, Approaches, and Innovations', in: *Plague in Antiquity*, ed. L. Hitchcock, A. Jamieson, and C. Tully, Ancient Near Eastern Studies Supplement Series (Leuven, Paris, and Walpole), 13–33

Attia and Buisson 2005 = A. Attia and G. Buisson, '[A.2025]: "un texte pour les médecins"', *Journal des Médecines Cunéiformes* 6, 41–42

Attia 2018 = A. Attia '"Mieux vaut être riche et bien-portant que pauvre et malade": de BAM III-234 à Job', *Journal des Médecines Cunéiformes* 31: 43–66

Bottéro 1978 = J. Bottéro, 'Antiquités assyro-babyloniennes', *École pratique des hautes études. 4e section, Sciences historiques et philologiques. Annuaire* 1977–1978, 107–164

Beckman 1997 = G. Beckman, 'Plague Prayers to Muršili II', in: *The Context of Scripture, Volume I: Canonical Composition from the Biblical World*, ed. W. W. Hallo and K. L. Younger (Leiden: Brill)

De Zorzi 2011 = N. De Zorzi, 'The Omen Series *šumma izbu*: Internal Structure and Hermeneutic Strategies', *KASKAL* 8, 43–75

Dossin and Finet 1978 = G. Dossin and A. Finet, *Correspondance féminine*, Archives royales de Mari 10 (Paris: Librairie orientaliste Paul Geuthner)

Dossin 1952 = G. Dossin, *Correspondance de Iasmaḫ-Addu*, Archives royales de Mari 5 (Paris: Librairie orientaliste Paul Geuthner)

Durand 1977 = J.-M. Durand, 'Notes sur l'histoire de Larsa (I)', *Revue d'Assyriologie* 71/1, 17–34

Durand 1988 = J.-M. Durand, *Archives Épistolaires de Mari 1/1*, Archives royales de Mari 26/1 (Paris: Librairie orientaliste Paul Geuthner)

Durand 2000 = J. M. Durand, *Les documents épistolaires du palais de Mari III*, Littératures Anciennes du Proche-Orient 18 (Paris: Les Éditions du Cerf)

Eidem 2011 = J. Eidem, *The Royal Archives from Tell Leilan. Old Babylonian Letters and Treaties from the Lower Town Palace East*, PIHANS 117 (Leiden: Nederlands Instituut voor het Nabije Oosten)

Esztári 2018 = R. Esztári, *Secrets from the Deep: Internal Structure and Systems of Interpretation in the Omen Series Šumma izbu* [PhD Dissertation] (Budapest)

Frankena 1966 = R. Frankena, *Briefe aus dem British Museum (LIH und CT 2–33)*, Altbabylonische Briefe in Umschrift und Übersetzung 2 (Leiden: Brill)

Freedman 2017 = S. M. Freedman, *If a City Is Set on a Height, The Akkadian Omen Series Šumma ālu ina mēlê šakin, Volume 3: Tablets 41–6*, Occasional Publications of the Samuel Noah Kramer Fund (Winona Lake: Eisenbrauns)

Geller 2010 = M. J. Geller *Ancient Babylonian Medicine: Theory and Practice* (Chichester: Wiley-Blackwell)

Goodnick-Westenholz 1983 = J. Goodnick-Westenholz, 'Review of Die altbabylonischen Briefe und Urkunden aus Kisurra by Burkhart Kienast', *Journal of Near Eastern Studies* 42, 219–228

Groneberg 1980 = B. Groneberg, *Die Orts- und Gewässernamen der altbabylonischer Zeit*, Répertoire Géographique des Textes Cunéiformes 3 (Wiesbaden: Dr. Ludwig Reichert Verlag)

Hallo 1976 = W. W. Hallo, 'The Royal Correspondence of Larsa: I. A Sumerian Prototype for the Prayer of Hezekiah?', in: *Kramer Anniversary Volume, Cuneiform Studies in Honor of Samuel Noah Kramer*, ed. B.L. Eichler, J.W. Heimerdinger, and Å.W. Sjöberg, Altes Testament und Alter Orient 25 (Neukirchen-Vluyn: Verlag Butzon und Bercker Kevelaer), 209–224

Hunger 1992 = H. Hunger, *Astrological reports to Assyrian kings*, State Archives of Assyria 8 (Helsinki: Helsinki university press)

Joannès 2022 = F. Joannès, '"Lorsqu'une épizootie s'y est déclarée . . ." (*Šibṭu kī ina libbi iššaknu*)', *le Journal des Médecines Cunéiformes* 39, 1–9

Leibovici 1956 = *M. Leibovici*, 'Un texte astrologique akkadien de Boghazköi', *Revue d'assyriologie et d'archéologie orientale* 50, 11–21

Leichty 1970 = E. Leichty, *The Omen Series Šumma Izbu* (Locust Valley: J. J. Augustin)

Livingstone 1989 = A. Livingstone, *Court Poetry and Literary Miscellanea*, State Archives of Assyria 3 (Helsinki: Helsinki university press)

Luukko 2012 = M. Luukko, *The Correspondence of Tiglath-Pileser III and Sargon II from Calah/Nimrud*, State Archives of Assyria 19 (Winona Lake: Eisenbrauns)

Maul 1999 = S. Maul, 'How the Babylonians Protected Themselves against Calamities Announced by Omens', in: *Mesopotamian Magic. Textual, Historical, and Interpretative Perspectives*, ed. T. Abusch and K. van der Toorn, Ancient Magic and Divination 1, (Groningen: Styx Publications), 123–129

Moran 1992 = W. Moran, *The Amarna Letters* (Baltimore: Johns Hopkins University Press)

Neumann et al. 2022 = G. U. Neumann, E. Skourtanioti, M. Burri, E. A. Nelson, M. Michel, A. N. Hiss, P. J. P. McGeorge, P. P. Betancourt, M. A. Spyrou, J. Krause, and P. W. Stockhammer, 'Ancient Yersinia pestis and Salmonella enterica genomes from Bronze Age Crete', *Current Biology* 32/16, 3641–3649

O'Brien 2013 = S. O'Brien, 'Communicable Disease Epidemics', in: *Oxford Handbook of Public Health Practice* [3rd edition], ed. C. Guest, W. Ricciardi, I. Kawachi, and I. Lang (Oxford: Oxford University Press), 166–177

Oppenheim 1977 = A. L. Oppenheim, *Ancient Mesopotamia. Portrait of a Dead Civilization* [Revised Edition completed by Erica Reiner] (Chicago/London: University of Chicago Press)

Oshima and Anthonioz 2023 = T. M. Oshima and S. Anthonioz, *Affronter le mal en Babylonie: théodicées akkadiennes*, Littératures anciennes du Proche-Orient 23 (Paris: Les Éditions du Cerf)

Parpola 1993 = S. Parpola, *Letters from Assyrian and Babylonian Scholars*, State Archives of Assyria 10 (Helsinki: Helsinki University Press)

Parpola and Watanabe 1988 = S. Parpola and K. Watanabe, *Neo-Assyrian Treaties and Loyalty Oath*, State Archives of Assyria 2 (Helsinki: Helsinki University Press)

Reiner 1958 = E. Reiner, *Šurpu: A Collection of Sumerian and Akkadian Incantations*, Archiv für Orientforschung, Beiheft 11 (Wien: Institut für Orientalistik der Universität)

Sachs and Hunger 1988 = A. J. Sachs and H. Hunger, *Astronomical Diaries and Related Texts From Babylonia. Volume I. Diaries from 652 B.C. to 262 B.C.* (Vienna: Verlag der Österreichischen Akademie der Wissenschaften)

Sachs and Hunger 1996 = A. Sachs and H. Hunger, *Astronomical Diaries and Related Texts from Babylonia. Volume III: Diaries from 164 B.C. to 61 BC* (Vienna: Verlag der Österreichischen Akademie der Wissenschaften)

Sasson 2017 = J. Sasson, *From the Mari Archives: An Anthology of Old Babylonian Letters* (Winona Lak: Eisenbrauns).

Singer 2017 = G. G. Singer, 'Beyong Amarna: "The Hand of Nergal" and the Plague in the Levant', *Ugarit-Forschunger* 48, 223–248

Singer 2021 = G. G. Singer, 'Peste Bubónica y Malaria en El Amarna', in: *Sociedades Antiguas del Creciente Fértil: Territorios, Memorias e Identidades Culturales*, ed. R.R. Rodríguez, Remitente Patagonia 3/1 (Buenos Aires: Remitente Patagonia), 51–74

Stol 1979 = M. Stol *On Trees, Mountains, and Millstones in the Ancient Near East*, Mededelingen en Verhandelingen Ex Oriente Lux 21, (Leiden: Ex Oriente Lux)

Stol 2009 = M. Stol, '"To Be Ill" in Akkadian: The Verb *salā'u* and the Substantive *sili'tu*', in: *Advances in Mesopotamian Medicine from Hammurabi to Hippocrates*, ed. A. Attia, G. Buisson and M. J. Geller, Cuneiform Monographs 37 (Leiden/Boston: Brill), 29–46

Wiseman and Black 1996 = D. J. Wiseman and J. A. Black, *Literary Texts from the Temple of Nabû*, Cuneiform Texts from Nimrud 4 (London: The British School of Archaeology in Iraq)

Ziegler 1999 = N. Ziegler, *Florilegium marianum IV. Le Harem de Zimrî-Lîm*, Mémoires de NABU 5 (Paris: SEPOA)

Ziegler and Langlois 2016 = N. Ziegler and A-I. Langlois, *Les toponymes paléo-babyloniens de la Haute-Mésopotamie*, Matériaux pour l'étude de la toponymie et de la topographie I/1 (Antony: SEPOA)

Eckart Frahm

Pandemic, Climate Change, and an Unknown Rebel King: Crisis and Empire in Mid-eighth Century BCE Assyria

For the Angel of Death spread his wings on the blast,
And breathed in the face of the foe as he passed;
And the eyes of the sleepers waxed deadly and chill,
And their hearts but once heaved, and for ever grew still!

(*Lord Byron*, The Destruction of Sennacherib)

The debate about where to locate the world's first empire will probably never be fully resolved. Some modern scholars have argued that empires are a fairly recent phenomenon, with beginnings around 1500 CE. Others, taking the opposite view, have traced the earliest empires in third and second millennium BCE western Asia and north-eastern Africa, in the kingdom of Akkad (c. 2350–2100 BCE), or Egypt's New Kingdom (c. 1550–1350 BCE). Still others consider Rome the first empire in history.[1]

What counts as an empire depends, of course, on how one defines the term. While there is an extensive debate about this question, certain criteria are widely accepted. Empires, it is generally assumed, are characterized by their considerable size;[2] the fact that they rule over areas that lie outside their original core territory; an osmotic imbalance between imperial centre and imperial periphery, with wealth being funnelled from the latter into the former; a great deal of ethnic, cultural, and religious diversity; and the application of both direct and indirect forms of governance.[3] If one uses the aforementioned benchmarks to assess whether the Mesopotamian (and Egyptian) states of the third and second millennium were actual empires, these seem all to fall somewhat short.[4] The kingdom of Akkad or Egypt's New Kingdom can certainly be called "aspirational empires",[5] but the imperial rhetoric used by their rulers did not yet translate into a tangible political reality.

In my view, the world's first state that became a "real" empire was the Neo-Assyrian kingdom of the first millennium BCE.[6] To be sure, the leading scholars and scribes of the Neo-Assyrian period never coined a specific term to define the new geopolitical entity that emerged during their time. But the Neo-Assyrian kingdom's massive size, complex organization, ethnic and religious diversity, and centralized yet at the same time flexible government structure justify calling it an empire. This was, at any rate, the way many writers of the Greco-Roman period, from the Greek historian Ctesias of Cnidus to the Roman Pompeius Trogus to the Late Antique Christian author Orosius, viewed the Neo-Assyrian state.[7]

Obviously, Assyria's imperial phase did not start right at the beginning of the Neo-Assyrian period. During the early stages of this era, in the later tenth and early ninth centuries BCE, Assyria's kings were focused on reconquering territories

1 The recent two-volume world history of empire by Bang, Bayly, and Scheidel (2021) begins its comprehensive historical survey with Egypt's Old Kingdom (not acknowledged as a full-scale empire, though) and the Akkad and Ur III states in Mesopotamia, both thriving in the second half of the third millennium BCE. For a critique of attempts to consider some of the world's earliest states empires, but also of "presentist" uses of the term, see Liverani 2017: 4–5

2 How large exactly a state needs to be to qualify as an empire is of course hard to determine. Each of the eighty-two historical empires listed by Scheidel 2021: 92–94 comprises at least one million square kilometres of land.

3 These are the main criteria set forth by Howe 2002: 14–15.

4 See Richardson 2020: 167: "The heroic word ['empire'] fits poorly on the skinny frames of Uruk, Ur, and maybe even Akkad: these states are either not large enough, long-lived enough . . . or internally coordinated enough to seem to fully qualify".

5 For this term, see Düring 2020: 8.

6 For more discussion, see Frahm 2023: 136–138.

7 For details, see Rollinger 2017.

Note: I have lectured on the topic of this paper at the universities of Oxford, Yale, Leipzig, Würzburg, and Heidelberg, and at the College of Arts in Baghdad. For the feedback I received at these different venues, in particular, of course, the Oxford conference that gave rise to the present volume, I am profoundly grateful. I have not significantly updated this article since submitting it in 2023. The "new" Tiglath-pileser discussed below will be covered in more detail, along with two other newly identified Neo-Assyrian kings, in a forthcoming study by Alexander Edmonds and the present author that will be published in the 2026 issue of the *Journal of Cuneiform Studies*.

Eckart Frahm, Yale University

 | https://doi.org/10.1515/9783112238622-005

Assyria had lost between 1050 and 950 BCE, when climate change, Aramaic migrations, and economic contraction had caused the Assyrian state to shrink dramatically. Even the reign of Shalmaneser III (858–824 BCE), when Assyria's "Reconquista"[8] had been completed and Assyrian armies began to venture into far-away regions all over Western Asia, cannot be characterized as "imperial", since these military forays hardly ever led to the permanent occupation of foreign lands.

It is only with the reign of Tiglath-pileser III (744–727 BCE) that Assyria's "imperialization" actually began. Annexing vast new territories and turning them into provinces headed by Assyrian governors,[9] Tiglath-pileser created a state that, by the end of his reign, comprised an area twice as large as the one he had inherited from his predecessor. There were other major changes as well. Prior to Tiglath-pileser's rise to power, Assyria's wealth had resulted to a significant extent from booty acquired during military campaigns, tribute received from vassal kings, and "presents" sent by political allies. Now, the "routinized plunder" of taxes, levied on people, livestock, crops, and trade and collected by the provincial governors, became an ever more important source of income for the Assyrian state.[10] Mass deportations on an unprecedented scale[11] contributed under Tiglath-pileser to a great deal of ethnic, linguistic, and religious diversity. A highly developed communication network based on well-kept roads and routinized information flows[12] and increased surveillance of potential troublemakers near and far[13] were additional factors in Assyria's transformation into what one can only describe as a true empire.

Numerous scholars have asked, sometimes almost obsessively, how this empire, for more than one hundred years so formidable and strong, could collapse so quickly, as it did in the years between 616 and 609 BCE.[14] Little attention, in contrast, has been paid to the opposite question, although it is no less puzzling: What brought about the birth of the Assyrian empire? Why was the reign of Tiglath-pileser III such a turning point? This essay will try to tackle this mystery, albeit without exploring it in the comprehensive manner only a more elaborate study could provide. It will argue that transmissible disease – the topic of the volume at hand – played an important role in the events at stake. But the reader is asked to be patient. Before the impact of plagues (and possibly also of climate change) on Assyria's history in the mid-eighth century BCE can be assessed in more detail, it is necessary to present a general outline of the political situation prior to Tiglath-pileser's reign – an outline that is based both on old and on new evidence.

***

The emergence of the Assyrian empire cannot be explained as the result of a gradual and steady rise experienced by the Assyrian state. In fact, the eighty years preceding Tiglath-pileser's accession were in many respects a time of crisis, especially for the Assyrian crown.

At first glance, the difficulties experienced by the ruling dynasty are not particularly obvious. The Assyrian King List, a key document for the reconstruction of the history of the Assyrian state, provides an unbroken sequence of rulers from one and the same family for the period from Shalmaneser III to Aššur-nerari V, Tiglath-pileser III's immediate predecessor:

102	Shalmaneser III (35)	858–824 BCE	son of Ashurnaṣirpal (II)
103	Šamši-Adad V (13)	823–811 BCE	son of Shalmaneser (III)
104	Adad-nerari III (28)	810–783 BCE	son of Šamši-Adad (V)
105	Shalmaneser IV (10)	782–773 BCE	son of Adad-nerari (III)
106	Aššur-dan III (18)	772–755 BCE	brother of Shalmaneser (IV)
107	Aššur-nerari V (10)	754–745 BCE	son of Adad-nerari (III)
108	Tiglath-pileser III (18)	744–727 BCE	son of Aššur-nerari (V)[15]

8 The application of this term to the history of Assyria goes back to Mario Liverani (see Liverani 2017: 119).

9 For the evolution of Assyria's provincial system during the Neo-Assyrian period, see Radner 2006.

10 For analysis, see Radner 2007.

11 For details, see now Sano 2020. All in all, Tiglath-pileser III's inscriptions claim that the king deported as many as 600,000 people during his reign, a number that is probably exaggerated, but not by that much.

12 See Radner 2014.

13 Frahm 2023: 268–272, and, for anonymous denunciations, Luukko 2018.

14 The French Assyriologist Paul Garelli famously called Assyria's fall "a historical scandal" (Garelli and Lemaire 1997: 123).

15 For an edition of the Assyrian King List, see Grayson 1980: 101–115. The number at the beginning of each entry indicates the position the respective king holds in the list, while that following his name in parentheses represents the number of years he ruled. King no. 108, Tiglath-pileser III, is only mentioned in the so-called SDAS List; the other manuscripts do not preserve this section. A text inscribed on bricks from

The impression of stability suggested by these entries is a mirage, however. The Assyrian kings of the late ninth and early eighth centuries did not enjoy happy and uncontested reigns. Several sources reveal that this was in many respects a perilous time for the dynasty. During the last years of Shalmaneser III and the first of Šamši-Adad V, a civil war involving various pretenders to the throne led to a situation in which, for several decades, historical actors other than the kings took centre stage. The most colourful of them was the royal consort and queen mother Sammu-ramat, who served as a regent during the early years of her son Adad-nerari III and later became the model of the famous Semiramis of Greek legend. Inscriptional evidence shows that Sammu-ramat, unique for a female member of the Assyrian royal family, even participated in – and possibly led – military campaigns.[16] But the Assyrian kings of the decades in question were not only side-lined by an unusually powerful woman – they also had to surrender much of their authority to a series of influential generals, provincial governors, and administrators, the so-called "magnates". These included Shalmaneser III's Field Marshal (*turtānu*) Dayyan-Aššur;[17] the provincial governor Nergal-ila'i, who later assumed the highest military rank as well; the Field Marshal Yaḫalu and the eunuch Palil-ereš; and most importantly, the Field Marshal Šamši-ilu. Installed by Adad-nerari III, the latter dominated Assyrian politics for some forty years, wielding power over western and eastern parts of the Assyrian state alike and commissioning several inscriptions in royal style, while the kings themselves left fewer and fewer such texts.[18]

For a long time, the rise of the "magnates" was considered by modern historians a phenomenon detrimental to the prosperity and integrity of the Assyrian kingdom. As the most recent scholar to espouse this view, A. Fuchs has compared the roles played by Sammu-ramat and Šamši-ilu to those of the "Empress Dowager" Cixi, who precipitated the fall of the Qing Dynasty in early twentieth century CE China, and of the military commander Flavius Stilicho, a man instrumental in bringing about the crisis of the Western Roman empire at the turn of the fourth to the fifth century CE.[19] Over the past decades, however, several other scholars, most notably S. Dalley, F. Blocher, and L. Siddall, have questioned this narrative of decadence.[20] Their argument has been that the "magnates" made good use of the autonomy they had acquired, promoting and furthering the economic development of the lands under their control. Such efforts would also have benefitted Assyria as a whole. In fact, archaeological surveys have shown that, starting in the late ninth century BCE, there was a substantial increase in settlements in the area between the Khabur, Euphrates, and Tigris Rivers, possibly as the result not only of more favorable climate conditions,[21] but also of sustained attempts by regional officials to convert parts of the steppe into agricultural land.[22] This supports the view that, at least initially, the impact the "magnates" had on the fortunes of the Assyrian state was more benign than has been traditionally assumed.

Yet it must also be stressed that things eventually changed. There can be no doubt that during the twenty-one years that passed from 765 to 745 BCE, Assyria suffered a massive crisis. This crisis had many facets. Most evident are its political manifestations. A key record for the period in question, otherwise poorly documented, is the Assyrian Eponym Chronicle, a text that lists for every year of the Assyrian calendar the official after whom that year was named, plus a particularly important historical event (occasionally also more than one) that had happened in its course.[23] Here is what the Eponym Chronicle has to say about the two decades preceding Tiglath-pileser III's reign:

765: to Ḫatarikka; plague (*mūtānu*) (reign of Aššur-dan III)
764: in the land
763: rebellion (*sīḫu*) in Libbi-ali (i.e., Ashur); solar eclipse in the month of Simanu
762: rebellion in Libbi-ali
761: rebellion in Arrapḫa

Ashur (Tadmor and Yamada 2011: Tiglath-pileser III, no. 58) claims that Tiglath-pileser III, rather than being a son of Aššur-nerari V, as the King List states, was a son of Adad-nerari III, an issue that will be discussed in more detail later.

16 See Siddall 2013: 86–100; Frahm 2016: 439–450.

17 In an inscription from Šadikanni on the Khabur, discussed and partly edited by Frahm 2015, it seems that Dayyan-Aššur (name restored) ascribes a number of military campaigns to himself rather than following the traditional practice of giving the king credit for them.

18 For historical analysis of the political and military roles these people played, see, inter alia, Grayson 1993 and Fuchs 2008. Mattila 2000 provides a systematic study of the Assyrian "magnates".

19 Fuchs 2008: 116, 125–126.

20 Dalley 2000, Blocher 2001, and Siddall 2013: 81–132.

21 Sinha et al. 2019.

22 See Bernbeck 2008, with earlier literature.

23 For an edition of the Neo-Assyrian eponym lists and chronicles, see Millard 1994.

760: rebellion in Arrapḫa
759: rebellion in Guzana; plague
758: to Guzana; peace in the land
757: in the land
756: in the land
755: to Ḫatarikka (accession of Aššur-nerari V)
754: to Arpad; return from Ashur (*issu* ^{uru}*aš-šur tayyārtu*)
753: in the land
752: in the land
751: in the land
750: in the land
749: to Namri
748: to Namri
747: in the land
746: rebellion in Kalḫu
745: On the 13th day of Ayyaru, Tukultī-apil-Ešarra (Tiglath-pileser III) ascended the throne.[24]

Usually, the event defining a given year in the Assyrian Eponym Chronicle was a military campaign conducted by the Assyrian king. But for the years between 765 and 746 BCE, the Chronicle lists only six such campaigns. In eight additional years, it claims that the king and his army stayed "in the land"; and for another six it records a "rebellion" in some Assyrian city: in Libbi-ali (that is, Ashur)[25] and Kalḫu in Assyria's core region, Arrapḫa in the east, and Guzana in the west. It is hence only too evident that all was not well in Assyria in the 760s, 750s, and 740s. Both internally and externally, the Assyrian state was facing massive challenges.

***

So far, the extent to which the authority of the ruling Assyrian monarchs was compromised during the fateful twenty-one years under discussion has been hard to gauge. Cuneiform documents shedding light on the events are few in number and not very rich in content.[26] But the darkness is not entirely impenetrable. A tablet known for more than one hundred years provides some intriguing new information on the crisis years. Poorly preserved as it is, there is little wonder that it has not yet been properly understood and has not received the attention it deserves.[27]

Housed in the British Museum under the accession number Rm 75, the tablet in question (see Fig. 1) seems to have been found at Nineveh, although (as will be argued further below) it was probably not drafted there. Only the upper right corner of its obverse and the corresponding lower right portion of its reverse are preserved. The fragmentary text inscribed on Rm 75 was published in the form of a cuneiform drawing (with restored signs added) by C. H. W. Johns in his ADD fascicle of 1898.[28] The first modern edition of the text appeared some seventy years later in J. N. Postgate's 1969 NARGD.[29] The most recent edition, largely identical with Postgate's, is found in L. Kataja's and R. Whiting's SAA 12 volume from 1995.[30]

24 Millard 1994: 40–43, 58–59.
25 For discussion of what "Libbi-ali" means in the two relevant entries in the Eponym Chronicle, see below.
26 Texts from Assyria from the time in question include two short and fragmentary royal building inscriptions from Ashur (see Grayson 1996: 245–247) and a treaty concluded between Aššur-nerari V and Mati'ilu of Arpad (Parpola and Watanabe 1988: no. 2). For archival documents, see the Munich "Archival Texts of the Assyrian Empire" (ATAE) project at http://oracc.museum.upenn.edu/atae/browsetextsbydate/index.html under "Ashur-dan III" and "Ashur-narari V" (the two most important texts from this group are discussed below, in n. 46 and 57). In a contemporary royal inscription from Urartu, the Urartian king Sarduri II claims to have defeated Aššur-nerari V at some point (Salvini 2008: 414–415, A 9–1, lato destro, lines 8–10). Inscriptions written in the names of the independent "governors"(?) of Suḫu on the Middle Euphrates (see Frame 1995: 275–331) cast some light on the political situation in mid-eighth century Mesopotamia as well; see Clancier 2021: 368–496 and Arbøll 2023: 65–69.
27 The main results of the following analysis have already been put forward, albeit very briefly, in Frahm 2023: 121, 127, 449 n. 4.
28 Johns 1898: no. 652.
29 Postgate 1969: no. 6.
30 Kataja and Whiting 1995: no. 13.

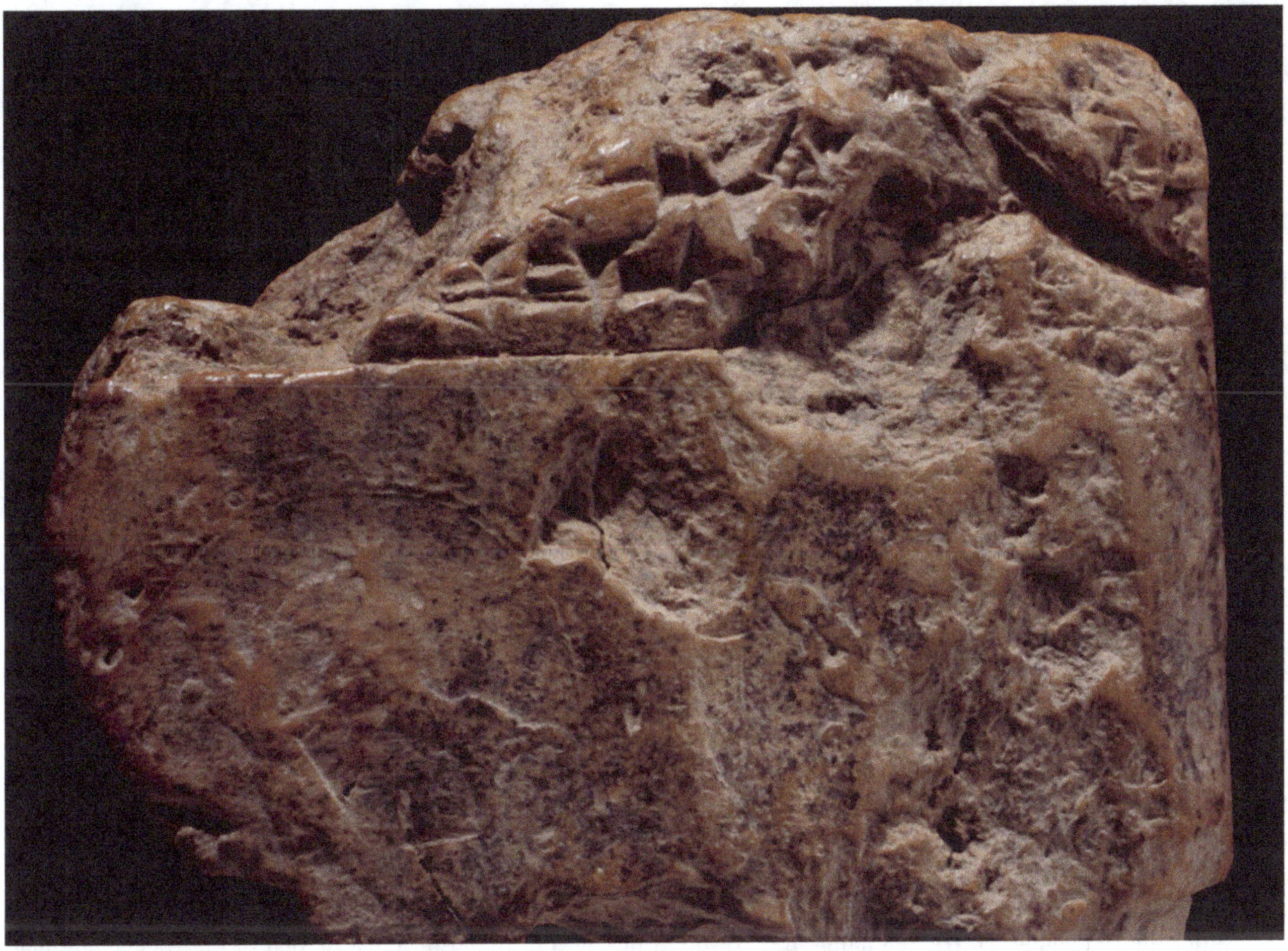

Figure 1: Rm 75, detail of the obverse (from https://cdli.mpiwg-berlin.mpg.de/dl/photo/P336253.jpg).

Despite the damage it incurred, it is clear that Rm 75 is a royal grant of a type well known from other Neo-Assyrian tablets.[31] The text begins with three very poorly preserved lines introducing the name and titles of the king issuing the grant. Ever since Johns's *editio princeps*, it has been assumed that the ruler mentioned here must have been Adad-nerari III. Based on a number of parallels, most notably the introductory passage of the royal grant K 310,[32] the passage has been restored by all of its previous editors as follows:

> [^{Id}IŠKUR–*né-ra-r*]*a* UGULA-*lum*
> [DUMU ^{I}*šam-š*]*i*–^{d}IŠKUR [UGULA]-*lum*
> [DUMU ^{Id}SIL]IM-*ma-nu*–M[AŠ UGULA-*lum-ma*]
>
> [Adad-nerar]i (III), overseer, [son of Šamš]i-Adad (V), [over]seer, [son of Sha]lmanes[er (III), likewise overseer].

The introductory lines of the tablet are followed by an uninscribed space with traces of two impressions of the Assyrian royal seal, showing the king in battle with a rampant lion.[33] The rest of the obverse and the upper portion of the reverse are lost. They must have provided specifics about the land granted and its recipient. When the text resumes towards

31 See Kataja and Whiting 1995: nos. 1–44.

32 Kataja and Whiting 1995: no. 10. The first three lines of this text read: ^{Id}IŠKUR–ERIM.TÁḪ LUGAL KUR *aš-šur* UGULA-*lum* / DUMU ^{I}*šam-ši*–^{d}IŠKUR LUGAL KUR *aš-šur* UGULA-*lum* / DUMU ^{Id}SILIM-*ma-nu*–MAŠ LUGAL KUR *aš-šur-ma* UGULA-*lum-ma*, "Adad-nerari (III), king of Assyria and overseer, son of Šamši-Adad (V), king of Assyria and overseer, son of Shalmaneser (III), likewise king of Assyria and overseer".

33 A third impression that must have been present on the left side of the sealing space (as seen again on K 310) is lost. One of the earliest testimonies to the use of the classical royal stamp seal in Neo-Assyrian times, the impressions on Rm 75 are catalogued as no. 5 in Mitchell and Searight 2007; see also Nadali 2009–2010: 235.

the bottom of the reverse, it talks about tax exemptions for the beneficiary of the grant, and then mentions the name of one Tiglath-pileser (Tukultī-apil-Ešarra),[34] whom Postgate as well as Kataja and Whiting identify as Tiglath-pileser III.[35] The text continues with a statement that the land granted should remain forever in the possession of its new owner – an otherwise unknown individual by the (probably West Semitic) name of Sa-abu[36] – and his descendants. Then follows an invocation of the deities Ashur, Adad, Ber, and Ištar-aššuritu, who are to guarantee that a later ruler (*rubû*) never revise the stipulations of the grant. The tablet ends with a date formula. Though again poorly preserved, it is clear that the eponym mentioned in it served in the year 762 BCE.[37]

Although basically accepted by all scholars who have studied the text since the days of Johns, there is a major problem with this reconstruction: the chronology seems all wrong. How can a royal grant issued by Adad-nerari III, who ruled from 810 until his death in 783 BCE, mention Tiglath-pileser III, who ruled from 744 to 727 BCE and probably didn't receive the name he bore as king prior to his accession to the throne? And how can the same grant, to make matters worse, be dated to 762 BCE? Something is seriously off here.

Previous attempts to resolve these issues have not really been successful. In the most recent discussion of the text, Kataja and Whiting, drawing on earlier remarks by Postgate, write:

> The dating of [text] no. 13 remains an enigma. The fact that Tiglath-pileser III is known to have been governor of Kalḫu before he became king gives a basis for connecting the style with [texts] nos. 6–8, which name a provincial governor in the text. But the date of 762 B.C., which seems probable, is still 20 years after the death of Adad-nerari III whose titles and genealogy appear at the beginning of the tablet.[38]

The authors essentially acknowledge that they are at a loss to explain the conundrum they are dealing with. Their claim that Tiglath-pileser III served as governor of Kalḫu prior to his reign as king is, moreover, poorly founded. The only reason why Forrer – who suggested this scenario more than a hundred years ago[39] – came up with it in the first place is that the rebellion that apparently brought Tiglath-pileser to power took place in Kalḫu[40] – all in all not a very strong argument.

Fortunately, there is a straightforward solution for all the problems at hand: one simply needs to give up the idea that the grant recorded in Rm 75 was issued in the name of Adad-nerari III. In fact, the name of this king, restored by all previous editors of the text in obv. 1 as [^{Id}IŠKUR–*né-ra-r*]*a*, is elsewhere never written in this way. Its second element, the word *nērārī* ("my support"), is usually rendered as ERIM.TÁḪ and in some cases, including a royal grant from the reign of Sargon II,[41] as *né-ra-ri*. A writing with final *ra*, which would be grammatically awkward, is nowhere attested.[42]

Rather than Adad-nerari III's, the name to be restored in obv. 1 of the grant must be that of the ruler mentioned again in rev. 3': Tiglath-pileser. I suggest reading the beginning of Rm 75 as follows:

> [^{I}*tukul-ti*–A–*é-šár-r*]*a* UGULA-*lum*
> [DUMU ^{I}*šam-š*]*i*–^{d}IŠKUR [UGULA]-*lum*
> [DUMU ^{Id}SIL]IM-*ma-nu*–M[AŠ UGULA-*lum-ma*]
>
> [Tiglath-piles]er, overseer, [son of Šamš]i-Adad (V), [over]seer, [son of Sha]lmanes[er (III), likewise overseer].

---

34 Postgate and Kataja and Whiting read the signs in rev. 3' as [. . .] $^{I\text{-}[\text{giš}]}$⸢*tukul*⸣-*ti*–A–*é-šár-ra*. According to Johns's copy, one could also read [. . .] ^{I}⸢*tukul*⸣-*ti*–A–*é-šár-ra*, which may, in fact, be slightly more likely. On the CDLI photo of the tablet at https://cdli.mpiwg-berlin.mpg.de/artifacts/336253/reader/167429, it is hard to make out the sign traces at the beginning of the name.

35 As a glance at the entry in PNA (Baker 2011) reveals, "Tukultī-apil-Ešarra" is attested only as a royal name: no commoners from the Neo-Assyrian period are known to have carried it. According to a Late Assyrian legal document (Kataja 1987), it was a punishable offense for commoners to give their children the names of certain kings.

36 ^{I}*sa-a-bu* DUMU ^{I}*a-ḫi*–^{d}*na-na*. For the interpretation of the first name as "(The deity) Sa is (my) father", see Kessler and Zadok 2002. Both the reading and interpretation of the name of Sabu's father remain uncertain; its understanding as Aḫī-Nanāya, "(The goddess) Nanaya is my brother", tentatively and not without misgivings proposed by Berlejung 1998, cannot be considered as definitive, not least because Nanaya is female.

37 The eponym in question, Ṭab-Bel, is said in the grant to have been [governor of] Bit-Zamani ($^{\text{rev. 11'}}$ [. . .] ^{I}DÙG–EN / $^{12'}$ [. . .] ⸢É⸣–*za-ma-ni*). The Assyrian Eponym Chronicles and Eponym Lists claim that Ṭab-Bel was governor of Amedu (see Millard 1994: 41), which seems at first glance not to align with the title he bears in the grant; but note that Amedu was the capital of the Assyrian province of Bit-Zamani.

38 Kataja and Whiting 1995: XXIV.

39 Forrer 1920: 10. Since Forrer put it forward, the completely conjectural idea that Tiglath-pileser had once served as governor of Kalḫu has been repeated so many times that it eventually became – as in the aforementioned statement by Kataja and Whiting – an unequivocal "fact".

40 As explicitly stated in the Assyrian Eponym Chronicle in the entry for 746 BCE, quoted above.

41 Kataja and Whiting 1995: no. 19, obv. 34'.

42 See Oded, Radner, and Brinkman 1998.

What this means is that in 762 BCE, a previously unknown Assyrian prince, who was a son of Šamši-Adad V[43] and grandson of Shalmaneser III, issued royal grants and decrees after assuming the royal name Tiglath-pileser.[44] In other words, we can add an additional Assyrian "king" to the many others already known.

The fact that the Assyrian King List fails to mention such a ruler for the year in question seems, at first glance, to undermine the scenario just outlined. But the Assyrian Eponym Chronicle provides additional evidence for it.[45] As already seen, the Chronicle states that in 763 and 762 BCE, a rebellion (*sīḫu*) had taken place in Libbi-ali, a well-known sobriquet for Ashur.[46] This lines up perfectly with the revised reading suggested for the grant text, which, even though apparently excavated at Nineveh, was most likely drafted at Ashur: the deities invoked in the text's final section, Ashur, Adad, Ber, and in particular *Ištar aššurītu*, the "Ištar of the city of Ashur", indicate as much.[47]

More corroboration of what is suggested here comes from K 51, one of the manuscripts of the aforementioned Eponym Chronicle; in Millard's edition it bears the label B1.[48] On this tablet, horizontal rulings precede, as a rule, references to (new) kings;[49] but there is also a ruling after the entry for the year 764 BCE – which is not followed by a royal name. Only one viable explanation for the presence of this ruling comes to mind: some now lost manuscript(s) of the Assyrian Eponym Chronicle must have included a note on Tiglath-pileser assuming royal power in 763 BCE – and even though the name of the usurper king was later cleansed from the record, we have to assume that the ghostly ruling continued to remind attentive readers of his one-time tenure and the dramatic events of 763/762. Notably enough, K 51 was found in Sennacherib's Southwest Palace at Nineveh,[50] suggesting some kind of official acknowledgement of the new Tiglath-pileser even outside the confines of Ashur.[51]

What happened in 763 BCE in the age-old centre of Assyrian religion now becomes much clearer. A son of Šamši-Adad V, probably filled with disgust about the ineffective rule of his nephew, Aššur-dan III, started a rebellion against

---

43 His mother may have been the formidable Sammu-ramat, Šamši-Adad's main consort, even though this is of course not certain.

44 The passage in rev. 3'–4' that mentions him again probably states that Tiglath-pileser swore an oath promising to keep the conditions of the grant in place. Based on a possible parallel in Kataja and Whiting 1995: no. 85, rev. 19, the following reconstruction suggests itself: [. . .] ^{I}⸢*tukul*⸣*-ti–A–é-šár-ra* / [*šarru/uklu nīš ili izakkar a*]*-na* EGIR *u*$_4$*-me*, "Tiglath-pileser, [the king/overseer, will take an oath that i]n the future . . ." (but cf. also Kataja and Whiting 1995: no. 14, rev. 2'–3').

45 Note that there might be yet another Middle/Neo-Assyrian ruler whose name is not included in the Assyrian King List. VAT 10136 (Frahm 2009: no. 22), a votive inscription on a clay tablet from Ashur, credits in line 7 a certain Ashur-uballiṭ with the restoration of a libation vessel dedicated to the god Ashur. This must have happened at some point between the reigns of Tukulti-Ninurta I (c. 1243–1207 BCE), who commissioned the vessel, and Tukulti-Ninurta II (890–884 BCE), whose craftsmen worked on it later. The text does not provide Ashur-uballiṭ with a title, royal or otherwise, but his name, only rarely attested for commoners, seems to suggest that he was a king, although possibly only acknowledged (probably for a short period of time) in Ashur.

46 Fuchs (2008: 86) argues that the toponym Libbi-ali in the Chronicle entries for 763 and 762 BCE refers to the citadel of Kalḫu rather than the city of Ashur. He hypothesizes that the Assyrian court under Aššur-dan III was evacuated from Kalḫu in 763 BCE, presumably by the powerful Field Marshal Šamši-ilu, moved to Ashur, and returned from there only in 754 BCE, in the first regnal year of Aššur-dan III's successor Aššur-nerari V. The court's homecoming, Fuchs claims, is suggested by the Chronicle entry for that year, *issu* ^{uru}*aš-šur tayyārtu*, "return from Ashur". But this hypothesis is fraught with difficulties and in my view unlikely. Libbi-ali is an extremely well-established term for Ashur, especially the temples and palaces in the northern part of the city. In an entry for the year 716 BCE in one of the eponym lists, it clearly refers to Ashur and not to Kalḫu (see Millard 1994: 47). Using it for the latter in the entries for 763 and 762 BCE would have caused massive confusion to any ancient reader of the Eponym Chronicle. What is more, a document from Kalḫu dated to the month of Tashritu (VII), 762 BCE (Ahmad and Postgate 2007: no. 29), belongs to the archive of a eunuch of the chief administrator of the household of the queen, which strongly suggests that Aššur-dan III's royal court was present in Kalḫu in the year in question (see also Ahmad and Postgate 2007: no. 53). Which event lies behind the enigmatic "return from Ashur" recorded for the year 754 remains for the time being unclear. The entry does not claim that the destination of the returnees was the city of Kalḫu and may in fact not refer to the king and his court at all.

47 See Meinhold 2009: 51–116, esp. 52.

48 For a hand copy, see Millard 1994: Plate 11–12.

49 As observed by Millard (1994: 13), the ruling after the entry for Bel-dan, eponym of the year 734 BCE, is a scribal mistake; it should have ruled off the entry for the previous term of Bel-dan, in 744 BCE, which is followed by the eponymate of Tiglath-pileser III.

50 It is known for sure that the tablets with the numbers K 1 to K 278 were all discovered by Layard in the area of Rooms XL and XLI of that palace; see Reade 1986: 213.

51 I owe the observation about the ruling in B1 to Alexander Edmonds, who has found additional indirect evidence for the upheavals of 763/762 in the Eponym List SU 52/150 from Sultantepe, Millard's manuscript A8. Edmonds will present the complex arguments bolstering his new interpretation of that list in a forthcoming publication.

the latter. His goal was to become king himself.[52] To bolster his ambitions, he took on the royal name Tiglath-pileser, most likely with the goal of placing himself in the tradition of the great late Middle Assyrian king Tiglath-pileser I.[53]

The rebel king and his supporters may have found encouragement for their uprising in a famous celestial event, which is mentioned in the Assyrian Eponym Chronicle's entry for 763 BCE alongside the rebellion in Ashur: the solar eclipse of June 15, which has served as the backbone of first millennium BCE Mesopotamian chronology for more than 150 years.[54] It is the only such observation recorded in the Chronicle, a clear indication of the impact it had at the time on the collective psyche of the Assyrians. The citizens of Ashur may well have believed that, with the eclipse, the moment had come for the demise of the ruling king and the rise of a "Prince of Darkness". After all, as a cuneiform astrological omen told them, "[If in the month of Simanu[55] (a solar eclipse takes place), the king will die and a son of the kin]g will seize the throne".[56]

The tenure of the rebel king Tiglath-pileser in Ashur seems to have come to an end in 762 BCE, under circumstances that remain largely unknown.[57] But in the following years, other rebellions broke out in Arrapḫa and Guzana, undoubtedly contributing to an even greater degree of political instability.[58] Whether our Tiglath-pileser was involved in them is unclear. It cannot be excluded that he managed to escape from Ashur in 762 BCE and continued his quest for the crown first further east and then in the west; but positive evidence for such a course of events is lacking.[59] Be this as it may, the Assyrian kings residing in Kalḫu must have been under enormous pressure. As indicated by the Eponym Chronicle, the chaotic situation lasted until 745 BCE, weakening the internal fabric of the state and bringing Assyria's mission to expand into new regions to a temporary stall.

***

52 This seems to be the case despite the fact that the introductory lines of Rm 75 call him "overseer" (*uklu*) rather than "king" (*šarru*). In Neo-Assyrian royal grants and decrees, legal documents par excellence, *uklu* was the proper way to identify the ruler, whereas the title *šarru* is found only in exceptional cases, such as K 310 (Kataja and Whiting 1995: no. 10). Note, moreover, that Rm 75, as pointed out above, bears impressions of the Assyrian royal seal.

53 As discussed by Frahm 2005, all Assyrian kings who ruled from the late eleventh century to the reign of Shalmaneser V (726–722 BCE) used throne names harking back to famous Middle Assyrian forebears. Alternatively, one could speculate that Tiglath-pileser III assumed his royal name in honour of the rebel king of 763/762 – both rulers, after all, ascended the throne in the wake of rebellions.

54 For a defence of the traditional dating of the solar eclipse mentioned in the Eponym Chronicle, see Hunger 2008.

55 This is the month during which, according to the Eponym Chronicle, the 763 eclipse took place; see above.

56 [DIŠ *ina* ^{iti}SIG$_4$ LUGAL ÚŠ-*ma* DUMU LUG]AL AŠ.TE DAB-*bat* (K 2208+, obv. 3; see Fincke 2014: 138, 141). The notion that a solar eclipse bodes ill for ruling kings is widespread and also found in completely different contexts, for example in the writings of John Milton: ". . . as when the sun new risen / Looks through the horizontal misty air / Shorn of his beams, or from behind the moon / In dim eclipse disastrous twilight sheds / On half the nations, and with fear of change / Perplexes monarchs . . . " (Milton, *Paradise Lost* I 594–599).

57 Donbaz and Parpola 2001: no. 234, a legal document from Ashur dated to the 29th day of the month of Shabaṭu (XI), 762 BCE (or 859 BCE, but this seems much less likely), records the sale of a house to a member of the household of the Assyrian "Field Marshal" (*turtānu*), with another member of that household serving as a witness. The text seems to suggest that Shamshi-ilu, who held the office of "Field Marshal" at the time in question, was present in Ashur during the last months of 762, and could indicate that he played a role in removing the usurper king Tiglath-pileser from his position. There remains a lot of uncertainty, however. Most likely, the Tiglath-pileser who established himself in Ashur in 763 and 762 BCE is not to be identified with the later king Tiglath-pileser III, but the matter is not absolutely clear. An appendix at the end of this essay will discuss it in more detail.

58 Archaeological evidence from Guzana suggests that the Governor's Palace in that city was rebuilt in the mid-eighth century or slightly later. Some scholars have argued that the palace might have been wrecked during the revolt of 759 or its suppression one year later, but so far, no indications of a destruction by fire or a violent dismantling of the building have been discovered. For discussion, see Novák et al. 2021: 373–374.

59 Tadmor and Yamada 2011: Tiglath-pileser III, no. 2006, an unprovenanced brick inscription brought to my attention by Alexander Edmonds, records that a certain "Kiditê, provincial governor [of . . .] and Arrapḫa, protégé of Tiglath-[pileser]", dedicated some object or space related to a palace to "Tiglath-pileser ($^{I\text{-}giš}$*tukul-ti*–A–[*ešarra*]) [. . .], king of the lands (*šar mātāti*) [. . .]". Which Tiglath-pileser is referenced here is not immediately clear. At first glance, the benefactor's association with Arrapḫa could be taken as providing a link with the insurrection that occurred there in 761 and 760 BCE, in the immediate aftermath of the revolt in Ashur. All in all, though, considering, on one hand, that the ambitious royal title seems far too grand for our rebel king, and on the other, that names similar to Kiditê are so far only attested in Kassite and (late) Middle Assyrian texts (see Tadmor and Yamada 2011: 169), it seems decidedly preferable to date the brick inscription to the reign of Tiglath-pileser I. An additional argument against ascribing the text to Tiglath-pileser III is the fact that the governors of Arrapḫa in 745 and 735 BCE, respectively, were Nabû-belu-uṣur and Aššur-šallimanni, rather than Kiditê (see Millard 1994: 43–44, 59).

Any serious anatomy of a historical crisis needs to establish, first and foremost, what actually happened. But the structural or systemic factors that might have been the root causes of the events under study must be investigated as well. This does not mean that historians are forced to give up on the idea that the achievements or failings of "great men" (and women) can have a real impact too. In the case of the Assyrian crisis of the mid-eighth century, the actions of military leaders like the Field Marshal Šamši-ilu – and the corresponding inaction of the contemporary Assyrian kings – may well have been important drivers of the changes that took place.[60] But at the same time, there is evidence that other, perhaps greater forces played a role too.

One of these forces may have been climate change. A recent scientific study has shown that Assyria experienced during the mid-eighth century a slow decrease in the annual precipitation that was so vital for its agricultural output.[61] The beginnings of the so-called "Assyrian megapluvial" (a period of abundant rainfall) around 925 BCE had coincided with Assyria's political recovery following the massive crisis that had hit the kingdom between 1050 and 950 BCE. But by about 770 BCE, rainfall became again less plentiful. Man-made ecological degradation caused additional stress. Assyrian hunting expeditions decimated the elephant herds that used to be at home in Syria, and the ambitious building projects undertaken by Assyrian kings, plus their need for firewood for smelting iron ore, led to a gradual depletion of the region's forests.[62]

It is not quite certain, though, to what extent these developments really affected the Assyrian agrarian economy at the time. By the mid-eighth century, if one is to believe the aforementioned study, no massive droughts were yet in sight.[63] Something else, however, clearly did impact the situation in Assyria: plague.

The Assyrian Eponym Chronicle lists two outbreaks of epidemics for the period under discussion here: a first in the wake of a military campaign to Ḫatarikka in 765 BCE, and a second in 759 BCE, a year that also saw a rebellion in Guzana.[64] Since neither the Eponym Chronicle nor any other sources provide additional information on these outbreaks, many questions regarding them must remain open. But there is every reason to believe that they were highly disruptive and traumatizing events.

Widespread epidemics did apparently not occur all that often in Neo-Assyrian times. The only other year for which the Assyrian Eponym Chronicle records one is 802 BCE.[65] The Babylonian Chronicle documents an additional outbreak of plague in Assyria for the year 707 BCE.[66] Finally, beginning with the Jewish historian Josephus, it has been argued that the Biblical story about the "Angel of the Lord" putting to death overnight 185,000 of the Assyrian troops besieging Jerusalem during Sennacherib's western campaign of 701 BCE[67] may be a veiled reference to yet another epidemic, one that decimated the Assyrian army; but the evidence for such a scenario remains inconclusive.[68]

The nature of the infectious diseases that struck Assyria on the aforementioned occasions is nowhere specified. The Eponym Chronicle refers to them in all instances with the word *mūtānu*, which literally means "mass death". Like the Greek word Λοιμός and Latin *pestis*, *mūtānu* is a generic term that provides no clue regarding the kind of illnesses to which it is applied.[69] The fact that the Chronicle entries about plague outbreaks, in contrast to entries about revolts, fail to link these outbreaks to specific cities suggests that the illnesses alluded to were indeed widespread, but in the absence of additional textual or paleopathological data, all attempts to assess their causes, progression, and outcomes must remain, at least for the time being, a matter of speculation.

---

60 As strongly emphasized by Fuchs 2008.

61 See Sinha et al. 2019. The paleoclimatic data used by the authors was retrieved by tracking the ratios of oxygen and uranium isotopes in two limestone stalagmites – so-called speleothems – from the Kuna Ba cave near the city of Sulaymaniyah in Iraqi Kurdistan, some 300 kilometres southeast of Nineveh. The results of the study seem to be supported by proxy data from other locations.

62 See Çakırlar and Ikram 2016 and Rosenzweig 2016.

63 It is hard to quantify, of course, from which point on more arid conditions begin to have a major effect on agricultural productivity. In the southern regions of Assyria's core, where rainfall was, in general, relatively scarce, even small fluctuations might have been significant.

64 See the translation of the Chronicle above.

65 See Millard 1994: 34, 57.

66 See Grayson 1975: 76, line 5'. As observed by Radner (2009: 230), this last epidemic is apparently also referenced in two letters from the correspondence of Sargon II from Western Syria, Parpola 1987: nos. 171 and 180, indicating how widespread it was.

67 2 Kings 19: 35; Isaiah 37: 36; 2 Chronicles 32: 21.

68 For discussion and earlier literature, see Frahm 2023: 205–209, 458.

69 For references to *mūtānu* in the Akkadian textual record, see CAD M/2: 296–297.

One such attempt has been made by K. Radner, who observed that the plague of 765 BCE is mentioned in the Eponym Chronicle along with an Assyrian military campaign to Ḫatarikka on the Orontes River in Syria. For Radner, these two events were possibly linked: when fighting in the swampy, mosquito-ridden marshes of the Orontes Estuary, Radner suggests, the Assyrian troops caught some arbovirus-induced illness and brought it home, where it was soon contracted by significant portions of the Assyrian population. Radner's identification of the illness as an arborvirus disease is based on texts from Late Bronze Age Ḫattuša that describe rituals against the outbreak of epidemics during military campaigns. These epidemics, the texts claim, caused the death not only of men, but also of horses and cattle – a typical feature of an arbovirus disease like West Nile Fever (which is passed on by mosquitoes from wild birds to horses and then to other domestic animals and human beings), but not an attribute of bubonic plague, malaria, or typhus.[70]

Whether the disease outbreak of 765 BCE affected both human beings and animals is unknown, of course, and Radner's reconstruction therefore uncertain. Another possibility is that the disease originated in Babylonia. In the years prior to 765, Assyrian troops operated on several occasions, in 771, 770, and 767 BCE, on Babylonian soil. Babylonia was in dire straits during this period. An inscription written in the name of Nabû-šumu-imbi, a governor of Borsippa, reveals that during the reign of Nabû-šumu-iškun (c. 761 to 748 BCE) the area of Borsippa was ravaged by "disorder, disturbances, revolt, and turmoil",[71] and there are hints that the situation under Nabû-šumu-iškun's predecessor Eriba-Marduk was not much better. Explicit evidence that the chaos in Babylonia was related to the outbreak of an infectious disease is missing, but one indirect clue for such a scenario does exist: the presumed composition date of the Babylonian Erra Epic.[72] Drawing on parallels between historical allusions found in the epic and specific events recorded in a variety of cuneiform sources for the reigns of Eriba-Marduk and Nabû-šumu-iškun, P.-A. Beaulieu has argued that Kabti-ilani-Marduk, the scholar credited in the Erra Epic with "authoring" the text, wrote it at some point during the decades leading up to the mid-eighth century BCE.[73] Rather than with epidemics, the epic deals with war and violence, but it refers to plague (*šibṭu*) at least once, if not a few more times.[74] This and the fact that all the mayhem described in the epic is blamed on Erra, the Mesopotamian plague god par excellence,[75] could indicate that plague was in fact a factor in the events informing the epic. Interestingly, at the end of the aforementioned inscription from Borsippa, Nabû-šumu-imbi draws on the Erra Epic (V 58) when expressing his wish that "by the [command(?)] of Erra, the raging one . . . , the sword of *plague* (*šibṭu*) shall not approach him, and safety be ordained for him".[76]

That the Assyrians contracted the infectious disease that would affect them so badly in the course of campaigns they conducted, in the late 770 and early 760s BCE, in Babylonia is of course, yet again, only speculation. All we know for sure, thanks to the entries in the Assyrian Eponym Chronicle, is that some epidemic ravaged Assyria in 765 and then again in 759 BCE. The two outbreaks were probably related, which means that the plague lingered in Assyria – and possibly outside of Assyria too – for at least half a dozen years. This must have caused great anxiety and hardship, not only in terms of public health, but also ideologically, politically, and economically.

Assyrian royal ideology implied that Assyrian kings, like the "rois thaumaturges" of the Middle Ages,[77] were able to cure people struck by plague. In a letter to Esarhaddon,[78] Itti-Šamaš-balaṭu, an Assyrian official based in Phoenicia, writes,

70 Radner 2009: 228–231. See also Parpola 1987: no. 171, a letter from the reign of Sargon II (see above, n. 66) that mentions the killing of a horse during a time of plague in the region of Ḫatarikka.

71 Frame 1995: 124, i 15'–17'.

72 Edition: Cagni 1969.

73 Beaulieu 2001. A similar composition date had already been proposed by von Soden (1971: 255–256), in part because of the epidemics recorded for the years 765 and 759 BCE in the Assyrian Eponym Chronicle.

74 Plague seems to be mentioned in Tablet V 53: *nāru ša iṣarraḫu ul imât ina šibṭi*, "The singer who (moanfully) chants (the epic) will not die from plague", and possibly also in V 58: *patar šibṭi ul iṭeḫḫēšū-(ma) šalimtu šaknassu*, "The sword of plague will not approach it (a house), and safety will be ordained for it", as well as in IV 76–77. The problem in all these cases is to determine whether the word used is really *šibṭu*, "plague" (which seems quite certain only in V 53), and not rather *šipṭu*, "judgment". For discussion, see Taylor 2017: 71–86.

75 Erra was closely associated with the Mesopotamian god Nergal, who in turn was associated with the Syrian god Resheph, the Greek god Apollo, and the Egyptian goddess Sekhmet (see Gestoso Singer 2017: 223–224). All these deities were considered agents of plague in ancient times.

76 Frame 1995: 126, ii 27'–28': *ina* [. . .] . . . *Erra šalbābi* . . . *patar* (*pat-ri*) *šibṭi lā iṭeḫḫēšu šalimtu šaknassu* (*šá-ak-na-si*). For a discussion of this passage and its dependence on Erra V 58 (quoted above in n. 74), see Taylor 2017: 74–77 (but note that Taylor prefers a reading *patar šipṭi*, "sword of judgment", over *patar šibṭi*, "sword of plague").

77 Bloch 1924.

78 Luukko and Van Buylaere 2002: no. 127.

"The king, my lord, has revived me from *a thousand* pestilences".[79] But such excesses of flattery had little to do with reality – and the failure of the kings to live up to them in case of actual need can only have further weakened their status.

In the absence of effective medical treatments, other means had to be taken to curb plague outbreaks. Documents from Old Babylonian Mari show that ancient Near Eastern authorities, just like those of modern times, tended to impose travel bans on such occasions. As a Mari letter specifies, "Inhabitants of the towns, as soon as they have been touched (by plague), must not enter untouched towns. Otherwise, it could well happen that they touch the whole country".[80] Most likely, similar measures were also implemented in mid-eighth-century Assyria – and one can easily imagine to what extent they must have paralyzed the kingdom's commercial life and military readiness, exacerbating a crisis that had already caused many people to die. It is all but certain that things were very bad.

***

And yet, at the end of the twenty-one *anni horribiles* the Assyrian kingdom experienced from 765 BCE onwards, another member of the Assyrian royal family, a man by the name of Pulu who called himself Tiglath-pileser (III) after becoming king, managed within just a few years not only to restabilize the Assyrian state, but also to massively expand it, effectively turning it into the world's first empire. In 746 BCE, he had started a revolt in Kalḫu; in 745 BCE, he ascended the Assyrian throne; and by the end of his reign, in 727 BCE, Assyria was the hegemon of much of Western Asia, from the Zagros Mountains in the east to the Mediterranean Sea in the west, and from the Anatolian highlands in the north to the Babylonian alluvial plain in the south. How is one to account for this almost miraculous transformation?

One factor that may have facilitated Assyria's rapid expansion under Tiglath-pileser III is rather obvious: while clear documentary evidence is unavailable, Assyria was quite possibly not the only country implicated by the plague outbreaks of the 760s and 750s. In neighbouring lands, the illness may have taken a heavy toll as well, which would have made it easier for Tiglath-pileser to conquer so many previously independent states within such a short time span.[81] To invoke a historical analogy: the so-called Justinian Plague, which broke out in Constantinople in 541 CE, caused the death of a significant portion of the people of Byzantium, but it also heavily affected populations in the west and the east of the Byzantine empire, enabling Justinian, despite the losses in life incurred at home, to eventually conquer all of Italy and parts of the western Mediterranean, and make peace with the Sasanians.[82] The situation in mid-eighth century Assyria may have been similar – it cannot be excluded that mortality rates in Assyria were actually lower than in adjoining territories.

Yet what is perhaps most important to take into consideration when thinking about the problem at hand is that history is not governed by deterministic rules. Challenges can be met by adapting to the changes taking place – at least up to a certain breaking point. That point had evidently not been reached when Tiglath-pileser III became king – neither climate change nor plague had delivered the death blow to the Assyrian state. And so, Tiglath-pileser had a chance to deal with the trials he faced.

He did so most successfully.[83] Taking stock of the losses of life the epidemics of the 760s and 750s had caused in the Assyrian heartland, and realizing that it was hard to boost crop production under increasingly unfavourable ecological conditions, the king decided to implement a new political strategy, one that focused on the conquest and annexation of

79 *i-na li-mu mu-ta-ni* LUGAL EN *ub-tal-*[*liṭ-a*]*-ni*. All scholars so far have taken *li-mu* in this sentence to represent the Akkadian word *līmu*, "thousand", and this is indeed the most likely interpretation. Still, one cannot entirely exclude the possibility that *li-mu* is actually a Greek gloss representing Λοιμός. After all, Itti-Šamaš-balaṭu wrote from a place not that far away from the site of Al-Mina on the Eastern Mediterranean, which was marked by a strong Greek presence.

80 Heimpel 2003: 184–185, Text 26 17. For reactions to plagues within the sphere of Mari and in Mesopotamia in general, see Farber 2004. The existence of rituals against plague in Assyria is documented by the "Manual of the Exorcist", known from copies from several Neo-Assyrian cities. This extensive catalogue of magical and medical texts and treatments includes a reference to procedures aimed at "dispelling *di'u*-disease, epidemic, and plague" (*di'u šibṭu mūtānu* (NAM.ÚŠ.MEŠ) *šūtuqu*); see Geller 2018: 299, line 20. A Neo-Assyrian cuneiform manuscript recording such procedures is KAR 298 (Wiggermann 1992: 41–103, text no. II), written by the eminent seventh century BCE exorcist Kiṣir-Aššur from Ashur. For the most recent discussion of this text, see Arbøll 2021: 138–143.

81 Note that Esarhaddon's Succession Treaty curses potential opponents of the Assyrian king and his crown prince by asking that "Nergal . . . send slaughter and pes[til]ence (*mu-t*[*a-a*]*-nu*) among you" (Parpola and Watanabe 1988: no. 6, line 456; see also line 480).

82 For an up-to-date account of the Justinian Plague and how it affected both the Mediterranean and Western Asia, see Harper 2017: 199–245. Note, too, as stressed by Sumption 1999: 51–101, that the plague epidemic of 1347–1350 CE, one of the greatest demographic catastrophes Europe ever suffered, did only briefly interrupt the Hundred Years War.

83 The following remarks draw on (and to some extent quote verbatim) Frahm 2023: 131.

foreign lands, the extraction of their wealth for the greater good of the Assyrian centre, and the deportation of hundreds of thousands of people from all areas of the newly expanded realm to gain the workforce needed to keep the state running. In addition, to make government processes more efficient, the king dismantled the decentralized power structure that had been in place under his predecessors, reserving all important decisions for himself. It was, all in all, a remarkable feat of political and demographic reengineering, possibly facilitated, as argued by Fuchs,[84] by the fact that Assyria's most powerful magnate, the Field Marshal Šamši-ilu, seems to have made sure in the years preceding Tiglath-pileser's accession that the Assyrian army remained ready and powerful, even though Šamši-ilu may have used it primarily for the inner-Assyrian conflicts in which he was engaged.

***

The hypothesis presented here may seem at first glance somewhat counter-intuitive. It flies in the face of the prevailing notion that pandemics and climate change bring about the fall rather than the rise of empires and civilizations – including our own. The Antonine Plague of 165–180 CE, the Plague of Cyprian some seventy later, and the Justinian Plague starting in 541 CE have been identified as major factors in the decline of the Roman Empire,[85] while the fall of the Khmer Empire in the fifteenth century CE and of the Maya civilization about half a millennium earlier have been attributed at least in part to climate change.[86] In the same vein, the recent study by Sinha et al. on climate change during the Neo-Assyrian period has tried to link the drought conditions that became more prevalent during the eighth and seventh centuries BCE in northern Mesopotamia to the demise of the Assyrian empire, and not its emergence.[87]

My hypothesis may also, for some, exemplify the perils of the "post-hoc fallacy" – the erroneous idea that an event that follows another was by necessity caused by it. After all, Tiglath-pileser III nowhere explicitly states that his aggressive new political program of annexation and deportation was initiated to compensate for the losses Assyria had suffered in the wake of the plague outbreaks of the previous two decades.

Still, at the very least, the ideas put forward in this article provide for the first time an attempt, to be scrutinized in future studies, to explain in a systematic way what triggered the dramatic changes brought about during Tiglath-pileser III's reign. The scenario outlined in the previous pages may also do something else: serve as a warning for our own times. For the Neo-Assyrian state was not a "nice" one. It achieved its imperialist goals through brutal conquest, calculated frightfulness, and political blackmail. The story told in this essay thus offers an illuminating example of how "bad actors" can take advantage of some of the major disasters, from climate change to pandemics, that tend to befall humanity. We better be on the lookout.

Appendix: "Tiglath-pileser 2.5" – on the identity of the rebel ruler of 763/762 BCE

The fragmentary royal grant earlier discussed in this article, Rm 75 (Kataja and Whiting 1995: no. 13), was apparently written on behalf of a so-far unknown rebel king who came to power in Ashur in 763 BCE, assumed the royal name Tiglath-pileser (Tukultī-apil-Ešarra), and was recognized as king in Assyria's old religious centre until the following year. Is there any chance that this man is to be identified with the Assyrian monarch who took on the same royal name in 745 BCE and founded the Assyrian empire, that is, Tiglath-pileser III? As will be shown in the following, the answer to this question is most likely negative, but some uncertainty remains.

There are two main reasons why the two Tiglath-pilesers are probably not one and the same person. The most important is that the Tiglath-pileser of the grant claims to have been a son of Šamši-Adad V, while Tiglath-pileser III was

84 Fuchs 2008: 107.

85 For elaborate discussion, see Harper 2017.

86 See Weiss 2017, with contributions on the Maya civilization by Douglas J. Kennett and David A. Hodell, and on the Khmer by Roland Fletcher et al.

87 Sinha et al. 2019. For my own thoughts on the reasons for Assyria's fall, see Frahm 2023: 323–347.

apparently either a son of the previous king, Aššur-nerari V, as suggested by the Assyrian King List,[88] or of Adad-nerari III, as claimed in a short text inscribed in the name of Tiglath-pileser III himself on several bricks from Ashur.[89]

This does not settle the matter once and for all, however. It is unlikely (though not impossible) that the Tiglath-pileser who was in power in Ashur in 763/762 BCE would have given a false filiation in a text recording a royal grant. In the case of Tiglath-pileser III, though, there is some serious uncertainty about his family background. The Assyrian King List, where father–son succession is the rule, could simply have made up that Tiglath-pileser III was a son of his predecessor. The "low-profile" brick inscriptions from Ashur, in turn, are the only texts composed in Tiglath-pileser III's name that provide information about the king's father and may be inaccurate as well, even though this is less likely.

If one accepts, for argument's sake, that Tiglath-pileser III was actually a son of Šamši-Adad V, then there is a second problem. Even assuming that Tiglath-pileser III was born at the very end of Šamši-Adad V's reign, in 811 BCE, he would have been sixty-six years old when ascending the throne in 745 BCE and eighty-four at his death in 727 BCE. For a king who implemented so many revolutionary changes, this seems exceedingly old – although one should remember that the Babylonian king Nabonidus, another great innovator, was probably in his late seventies or even in his eighties when Babylon was conquered by the Persians in 539 BCE, while his mother, Adda-guppi, reached an age of over one hundred years.[90]

One indirect argument that might support the assumption of a possible identity between the two Tiglath-pilesers is that there is evidence for close ties between Tiglath-pileser III and the city of Ashur, a connection for which no fully satisfactory explanation has been found so far. According to the Babylonian King List A, both Shalmaneser V and his father Tiglath-pileser III belonged to a "Dynasty of Ashur" (BALA *bal-til*^{ki}), whereas their successors, Sargon II (in all likelihood a son of Tiglath-pileser III) and Sargon's son Sennacherib, are said to represent a "Dynasty of *Ḫa-bi*-GAL", probably a designation for the western land of Ḫanigalbat (or Ḫanirabbat).[91] Tiglath-pileser is, moreover, the first Assyrian king to bear the royal epithet *pere' Baltil šūquru*, "precious scion of Baltil (i.e., Ashur)", later also assumed by Sargon II and other rulers.[92] It is, admittedly, pure speculation, but could this designation harken back to an attempt by Tiglath-pileser, made in 763 BCE, to establish himself as king in the city of Ashur? If so, this attempt would have come to naught, and the rebel ruler would have had to escape to the west, perhaps to the area around the city of Ḫarran, a region vaguely labelled as ḪaniGALbat, where Sargon, and eventually perhaps also Sennacherib, would have been born.[93] It cannot even be ruled out that Sargon, whose birth is usually dated to the 760s,[94] was born in Ashur during the years of the rebellion, and received his name, Šarru-ukīn, that is, "(DN) has firmly established the king", with reference to the royal ambitions his father Tiglath-pileser harboured during this time.[95]

Again, it should be stressed that the scenarios just outlined are extremely tenuous. But they are not impossible. It will require the discovery of new sources to determine if they should be rejected once and for all, or not.

Bibliography

Ahmad and Postgate 2007 = A. Y. Ahmad and J. N. Postgate, *Archives from the Domestic Wing of the North-West Palace in Kalḫu/Nimrud*, Edubba 10 (London: Nabu Publications)

Arbøll 2021 = T. Arbøll, *Medicine in Ancient Aššur: A Microhistorical Study of the Neo-Assyrian Healer Kiṣir-Aššur*, Ancient Magic and Divination 18 (Leiden: Brill)

Arbøll 2023 = T. Arbøll, *The Cuneiform Texts from the Danish Excavations of Ḥamā in Syria (1931–1938): Letters, Administrative Documents, Scholarly Texts, Inscriptions, and Seals* (Copenhagen: The Royal Danish Academy of Sciences and Letters)

88 For the relevant section of the King List, see above.

89 See Tadmor and Yamada 2011: Tiglath-pileser III, no. 58.

90 Schaudig 2001: 10–11, 14.

91 See Grayson 1980: 93.

92 See Tadmor and Yamada 2011: Tiglath-pileser III nos. 1:1, 35: i 23, and, for discussion, Tadmor 1981: 27–29.

93 For the close connections of the "Sargonids" with ḪaniGALbat and the city of Ḫarran, see May 2017; for an attempt to place greater emphasis on the importance that the western city of Dur-Katlimmu had for members of the Neo-Assyrian royal family, most notably Esarhaddon, see Jones 2023.

94 See Fuchs 2009: 53 and Frahm 2014: 175–176, both with earlier literature.

95 On Sargon II's name, see Frahm 2005 and Fuchs 2009: 51–53.

Baker 2011 = H. D. Baker, 'Tukultī-apil-Ešarra', in: *The Prosopography of the Neo-Assyrian Empire, Volume 3/II*, ed. H. D. Baker (Helsinki: The Neo-Assyrian Text Corpus Project), 1328–1331

Bang, Bayly, and Scheidel 2021 = P. F. Bang, C. A. Bayly, and W. Scheidel (eds.), *The Oxford World History of Empire, 2 volumes* (Oxford: Oxford University Press)

Beaulieu 2001 = P.-A. Beaulieu, 'The Abduction of Ištar from the Eanna Temple: The Changing Memories of an Event', in: *Historiography in the Cuneiform World*, ed. T. Abusch et al., CRRAI 45, Part I (Bethesda: CDL Press), 29–40

Berlejung 1998 = A. Berlejung, 'Aḫī-Nanāya', in: *The Prosopography of the Neo-Assyrian Empire, Volume 1/I*, ed. K. Radner (Helsinki: The Neo-Assyrian Text Corpus Project), 66

Bernbeck 2008 = R. Bernbeck, 'Sex/Gender/Power and Šammuramat: A View from the Syrian Steppe', in: *Fundstellen: Gesammelte Schriften zur Archäologie und Geschichte Altvorderasiens ad honorem Hartmut Kühne*, ed. D. Bonatz, R. M. Czichon, and F. J. Kreppner (Wiesbaden: Harrassowitz), 351–369

Bloch 1924 = M. Bloch, *Les Rois thaumaturges. Étude sur le caractère surnaturel attribué à la puissance royale particulièrement en France et en Angleterre* (Strasbourg: Istra)

Blocher 2001 = F. Blocher, 'Assyrische Würdenträger und Gouverneure des 9. und 8. Jh.: Eine Neubewertung ihrer Rolle', *Altorientalische Forschungen* 28, 298–324

Cagni 1969 = L. Cagni, *L'Epopea di Erra*, Studi Semitici 34 (Rome: Istituto di studi del Vicino Oriente dell'Università)

Çakırlar and Ikram 2016 = C. Çakırlar and S. Ikram, '"When Elephants Battle, the Grass Suffers": Power, Ivory and the Syrian Elephant', *Levant* 48, 167–183

Clancier 2021 = P. Clancier, *À l'ombre des grandes puissances de Mésopotamie: Une histoire du Sūhu à l'époque néo-assyrien*, Culture and History of the Ancient Near East 114 (Leiden: Brill)

Dalley 2000 = S. Dalley, 'Shamshi-ilu, Language and Power in the Western Assyrian Empire', in: *Essays on Syria in the Iron Age*, ed. G. Bunnens (Leuven: Peeters), 79–88

Donbaz and Parpola 2001 = V. Donbaz and S. Parpola, *Neo-Assyrian Legal Texts in Istanbul*, Studien zu den Assur-Texten 2 (Saarbrücken: Saarbrücker Druckerei und Verlag)

Düring 2020 = B. S. Düring, *The Imperialisation of Assyria* (Cambridge: Cambridge University Press)

Farber 2004 = W. Farber, 'How to Marry a Disease: Epidemics, Contagion, and a Magic Ritual Against the "Hand of the Ghost"', in: *Magic and Rationality in Ancient Near Eastern and Graeco-Roman Medicine*, ed. H. F. J. Horstmanshoff and M. Stol, Studies in Ancient Medicine 27 (Leiden: Brill), 117–132

Fincke 2014 = J. Fincke, 'The Seventh Tablet of the *Rikis Gerri* Series of *Enūma Anu Enlil*', *Journal of Cuneiform Studies* 66, 129–148

Forrer 1920: E. Forrer, *Die Provinzeinteilung des assyrischen Reiches* (Leipzig: J. C. Hinrichs)

Frahm 2005 = E. Frahm, 'Observations on the Name and Age of Sargon II, and on Some Patterns of Assyrian Royal Onomastics', *NABU* 2005, no. 44

Frahm 2009 = E. Frahm, *Historische und historisch-literarische Texte*, Keilschrifttexte aus Assur literarischen Inhalts 3 (Wiesbaden: Harrassowitz)

Frahm 2014 = E. Frahm, 'Family Matters: Psychohistorical Reflections on Sennacherib and His Times', in: *Sennacherib at the Gates of Jerusalem: Story, History, and Historiography*, ed. I. Kalimi and S. Richardson, Culture and History of the Ancient Near East 71 (Leiden: Brill), 163–222

Frahm 2015 = E. Frahm, '"Whoever Destroys This Image": A Neo-Assyrian Statue from Tell ʿAğāğa (Šadikanni)', *NABU* 2015, no. 51

Frahm 2016 = E. Frahm, 'Of Doves, Fish, and Goddesses: Reflections on the Literary, Religious, and Historical Background of the Book of Jonah', in: *Sibyls, Scriptures, and Scrolls: John Collins at Seventy*, ed. J. Baden, H. Najman, and E. J. C. Tigchelaar (Leiden: Brill), 432–450

Frahm 2023 = E. Frahm, *Assyria: The Rise and Fall of the World's First Empire* (New York: Basic Books)

Frame 1995 = G. Frame, *Rulers of Babylonia, from the Second Dynasty of Isin to the End of Assyrian Domination (1157–612 BC)*, Royal Inscriptions of Mesopotamia Babylonian Periods 2 (Toronto: University of Toronto Press)

Fuchs 2008 = A. Fuchs, 'Der Turtān Šamšī-ilu und die große Zeit der assyrischen Großen (830–746)', *Welt des Orients* 38 (2008), 61–145

Fuchs 2009 = A. Fuchs, 'Sargon II', in: *Reallexikon der Assyriologie und Vorderasiatischen Archäologie 12*, ed. M. Streck (Berlin: De Gruyter), 51–61

Garelli and Lemaire 1997 = P. Garelli and A. Lemaire, *Le Proche-Orient asiatique. Volume II: Les Empires mésopotamiens, Israël* [Third edition] (Paris: Presses Universitaires de France)

Geller 2018 = M. J. Geller, 'The Exorcist's Manual (KAR 44)', in: *Assyrian and Babylonian Scholarly Text Catalogues: Medicine, Magic and Divination*, ed. U. Steinert, Die babylonisch-assyrische Medizin in Texten und Untersuchungen 9 (Berlin: De Gruyter), 292–312

Gestoso Singer 2017 = G. Gestoso Singer, 'Beyond Amarna: The "Hand of Nergal" and the Plague in the Levant', *Ugarit-Forschungen* 48, 223–247

Grayson 1975 = A. K. Grayson, *Assyrian and Babylonian* Chronicles (Locust Valley, NY: J. J. Augustin)

Grayson 1980 = A. K. Grayson, 'Königslisten und Chroniken: B. Akkadisch', in: *Reallexikon der Assyriologie und Vorderasiatischen Archäologie 6*, ed. D. O. Edzard (Berlin: De Gruyter), 86–135

Grayson 1993 = A. K. Grayson, 'Assyrian Officials and Power in the Ninth and Eighth Centuries', *State Archives of Assyria Bulletin* 7, 19–52

Grayson 1996 = A. K. Grayson, *Assyrian Rulers of the Early First Millennium BC II (858–745 BC)*, Royal Inscriptions of Mesopotamia Assyrian Periods 3 (Toronto: University of Toronto Press)

Harper 2017 = K. Harper, *The Fate of Rome: Climate, Disease, and the End of Empire* (Princeton: Princeton University Press)

Heimpel 2003 = W. Heimpel, *Letters to the King of Mari*, Mesopotamian Civilizations 12 (Winona Lake: Eisenbrauns)

Howe 2002 = S. Howe, *Empire: A Very Short Introduction* (Oxford: Oxford University Press)

Hunger 2008 = H. Hunger, 'Zur Datierung der neuassyrischen Eponymenliste', *Altorientalische Forschungen* 35, 323–325

Johns 1898 = C. H. W. Johns, *Assyrian Deeds and Documents Recording the Transfer of Property . . . Chiefly of the 7th Century B.C., Volume 1* (Cambridge: Deighton, Bell and Co.)

Jones 2023 = C. W. Jones, 'Failed Coup: The Assassination of Sennacherib and Esarhaddon's Struggle for the Throne, 681–680 B.C.', *Journal of Ancient Near Eastern History* 10, 293–369

Kataja 1987 = L. Kataja, 'A Neo-Assyrian Document on Two Cases of River Ordeal', *State Archives of Assyria Bulletin* 1, 65–68

Kataja and Whiting 1995 = L. Kataja and R. Whiting, *Grants, Decrees and Gifts of the Neo-Assyrian Period*, State Archives of Assyria 12 (Helsinki: Helsinki University Press)

Kessler and Zadok 2002 = K. Kessler and R. Zadok, 'Sā-abu', in: *The Prosopography of the Neo-Assyrian Empire, Volume 3/I*, ed. H. D. Baker (Helsinki: The Neo-Assyrian Text Corpus Project), 1057

Liverani 2017 = M. Liverani, *Assyria: The Imperial Mission* (Winona Lake: Eisenbrauns)

Luukko 2018 = M. Luukko, 'Anonymous Neo-Assyrian Denunciations in a Wider Context', in: *Neo-Assyrian Sources in Context: Thematic Studies of Texts, History, and Culture*, ed. S. Yamada, State Archives of Assyria Studies 28 (Helsinki: The Neo-Assyrian Text Corpus Project), 163–184

Luukko and Van Buylaere 2002 = M. Luukko and G. Van Buylaere, *The Political Correspondence of Esarhaddon*, State Archives of Assyria 16 (Helsinki: Helsinki University Press)

Mattila 2000 = R. Mattila, *The King's Magnates: A Study of the Highest Officials of the Neo-Assyrian Empire*, State Archives of Assyria Studies 11 (Helsinki: The Neo-Assyrian Text Corpus Project)

May 2017 = N. N. May, 'The Vizier and the Brother: Sargon II's Brother Sīn-aḫu-uṣur and the Neo-Assyrian Collateral Branches', *Bibliotheca Orientalis* 74, 491–527

Meinhold 2009 = W. Meinhold, *Ištar in Aššur: Untersuchungen eines Lokalkultes von ca. 2500 bis 614 v. Chr.*, Alter Orient und Altes Testament 367 (Münster: Ugarit-Verlag)

Millard 1994 = A. R. Millard, *The Eponyms of the Assyrian Empire, 910– 612 BC*, State Archives of Assyria Studies 2 (Helsinki: The Neo-Assyrian Text Corpus Project)

Mitchell and Searight 2007 = T. C. Mitchell and A. Searight, *Catalogue of the Western Asiatic Seals in the British Museum. Stamp Seals III: Impressions of Stamp Seals on Cuneiform Tablets, Clay Bullae, and Jar Handles* (Leiden: Brill)

Nadali 2009–2010 = D. Nadali, 'Neo-Assyrian State Seals: An Allegory of Power', State Archives of Assyria Bulletin 18, 215–244

Novák et al. 2021 = M Novák, W. Orthmann, and J. Schmid, 'Das Gesamtergebnis der Ausgrabung des Palastes', in: *Tell Halaf: Der assyrische Statthalterpalast*, ed. A. Baghdo, L. Martin, M. Novák, and W. Orthmann, Tell Halaf VI (Wiesbaden: Harrassowitz), 353–377

Oded, Radner, and Brinkman 1998 = B. Oded, K. Radner, and J. Brinkman, 'Adad-nērārī', in: *The Prosopography of the Neo-Assyrian Empire, Volume 1/I*, ed. K. Radner (Helsinki: The Neo-Assyrian Text Corpus Project), 30–34

Parpola 1987 = S. Parpola, *The Correspondence of Sargon II, Part I: Letters from Assyria and the West*, State Archives of Assyria 1 (Helsinki: University of Helsinki Press)

Parpola and Watanabe 1988 = S. Parpola and K. Watanabe, *Neo-Assyrian Treaties and Loyalty Oaths*, State Archives of Assyria 2 (Helsinki: University of Helsinki Press)

Postgate 1969 = J. N. Postgate, *Neo-Assyrian Royal Grants and Decrees*, Studia Pohl (Series Maior) 1 (Rome: Pontificio Istituto Biblico)

Radner 2006 = K. Radner, 'Provinz. C. Assyrien', in: *Reallexikon der Assyriologie und Vorderasiatischen Archäologie 11*, ed. M. P. Streck (Berlin: De Gruyter), 42–68

Radner 2007 = K. Radner, 'Abgaben an den König von Assyrien aus dem In- und Ausland', in: *Geschenke und Steuern, Zölle und Tribute: Antike Abgabenformen in Anspruch und Wirklichkeit*, ed. H. Klinkott, S. Kubisch, and R. Müller-Wollermann, Culture and History of the Ancient Near East 29 (Leiden: Brill), 213–230

Radner 2009 = K. Radner, 'The Assyrian King and His Scholars: The Syro-Anatolian and the Egyptian Schools', in: *Of God(s), Trees, Kings, and Scholars: Neo- Assyrian and Related Studies in Honour of Simo Parpola*, ed. M. Luukko, S. Svärd, and R. Mattila (Helsinki: Finnish Oriental Society), 221–238

Radner 2014 = K. Radner, 'An Imperial Communication Network: The State Correspondence of the Neo- Assyrian Empire', in: *State Correspondence in the Ancient World: From New Kingdom Egypt to the Roman Empire*, ed. K. Radner (Oxford: Oxford University Press), 64–93

Reade 1986 = J. Reade, 'Archaeology and the Kuyunjik Archives', in: *Cuneiform Archives and Libraries*, ed. K. Veenhof, Compte rendu de la Rencontre Assyriologique Internationale 30 (Leiden: The Netherlands Institute for the Near East), 213–222

Richardson 2020 = S. Richardson, 'Because Empire Means Forever: Babylon and Imperial Disposition', in: *Short-term Empires in World History*, ed. R. Rollinger, J. Degen, and M. Gehler (Wiesbaden: Springer), 167–187

Rollinger 2017 = R. Rollinger, 'Assyria in Classical Sources', in: *A Companion to Assyria*, ed. E. Frahm (Malden: Wiley Blackwell), 570–582

Rosenzweig 2016 = M. S. Rosenzweig, '"Ordering the Chaotic Periphery": The Environmental Impact of the Neo-Assyrian Empire on Its Provinces', in: *The Provincial Archaeology of the Assyrian Empire*, ed. J. MacGinnis, D. Wicke, and T. Greenfield (Cambridge: McDonald Institute for Archaeological Research), 49–58

Salvini 2008 = M. Salvini, *Corpus dei testi Urartei. Volume I: Le iscrizioni su pietra e roccia – i testi* (Rome: Istituto di studi sulle civiltà dell'Egeo e del Vicino Oriente)

Sano 2020 = K. Sano, *Die Deportationspraxis in neuassyrischer Zeit*, Alter Orient und Altes Testament 466 (Münster: Ugarit-Verlag)

Schaudig 2001 = H. Schaudig, *Die Inschriften Nabonids von Babylon und Kyros' des Großen*, Alter Orient und Altes Testament 256 (Münster: Ugarit-Verlag)

Scheidel 2021 = W. Scheidel, 'The Scale of Empire: Territory, Population, Distribution', in: *The Oxford World History of Empire*, ed. P. F. Bang, C. A. Bayly, and W. Scheidel, Volume 1 (Oxford: Oxford University Press), 91–110

Siddall 2013 = L. R. Siddall, *The Reign of Adad-nīrārī III: An Historical and Ideological Analysis of an Assyrian King and His Times*, Cuneiform Monographs 45 (Leiden: Brill)

Sinha et al. 2019 = A. Sinha, G. Kathayat, H. Weiss, H. Li, H. Cheng, J. Reuter, A. W. Schneider et al., 'Role of Climate in the Rise and Fall of the Assyrian Empire', *Science Advances* 5, no. 11 (November)

Sumption 1999 = J. Sumption, *Trial by Fire: The Hundred Years War, Volume 2* (London: Faber and Faber)

Tadmor 1981 = H. Tadmor, 'History and Ideology in the Assyrian Royal Inscriptions', in: *Assyrian Royal Inscriptions: New Horizons*, ed. F. M. Fales (Rome: Istituto per l'Oriente), 13–33

Tadmor and Yamada 2011 = H. Tadmor and S. Yamada, *The Royal Inscriptions of Tiglath-pileser III (744–727 BC) and Shalmaneser V (726– 722 BC), Kings of Assyria*, Royal Inscriptions of the Neo-Assyrian Period 1 (Winona Lake, IN: Eisenbrauns)

Taylor 2017 = K. Taylor, *The Erra Song: A Religious, Literary, and Comparative Analysis* [PhD dissertation, Harvard University] (Cambridge)

Von Soden 1971 = W. von Soden, 'Etemenanki vor Asarhaddon nach der Erzählung vom Turmbau zu Babel und dem Erra-Mythos', *Ugarit-Forschungen* 3, 253–263

Weiss 2017 = H. Weiss (ed.), *Megadrought and Collapse: From Early Agriculture to Angkor* (Oxford: Oxford University Press)

Wiggermann 1992 = F. Wiggerman, *Mesopotamian Protective Spirits: The Ritual Texts*, Cuneiform Monographs 1 (Groningen: Styx)

3 Understanding and Conceptualizing Epidemics

Nils P. Heeßel

Comprehending Plague: The Late Babylonian Effort to Understand Epidemics

1 Sources for Epidemics in Mesopotamia

Compared to other fields of medical knowledge, we are quite well informed about epidemics in Mesopotamia, since epidemics are mentioned in a variety of sources, not only in medical texts. First and foremost, it is important to realise that the very basis of all epidemics, namely contagion, was not only well known but also a distinct concept in Mesopotamian thinking. The key evidence for this a passage in an Old Babylonian letter from king Zimri-Lim of Mari to his wife Šibtum:

> *eš-me-e-ma* ^{munus}*Na-an-na-mì si-im-ma-am mar-ṣa-at u it-ti* É.GAL-*lim ma-ga-al wa-aš-ba-at-ma* MUNUS.MEŠ *ma-da-tim it-ti-ša-ma i-sa-bi-ik i-na-an-na dan-na-tim šu-uk-ni-ma i-na ka-às i-ša-at-tu-ú ma-am-ma-an la i-ša-at-ti i-na* ^{giš}GU.ZA *ša úš-ša-bu ma-am-ma-an la úš-ša-ab ù i-na* ^{giš}NÁ *ša it-ti-il-lu ma-am-ma-an la it-te-e-el-ma* MUNUS.MEŠ *ma-da-tim it-ti-ša-ma la i-sa-ab-bi-ik* [*si-im-m*]*u-um šu-ú mu-uš-ta-aḫ-ḫi-zu*

> "I have heard that Nanna is suffering from a lesion; yet, she frequents the palace. It will infect many women with her (ailment). Now, then, give strict orders that no one drink from the cup she uses, and no one sit in the seat in which she sits, and no one lie on the bed in which she lies, so that it should not infect many women with her (ailment). That [lesi]on is a catcher."[1]

This often-cited letter shows clearly the knowledge of contagion and also of isolation as the means to overcome it. One may wonder, why it is important to stress this since contagion and isolation probably are known since the cognitive revolution of humankind. Yet, it is important to be clear about the Mesopotamians being very much aware of the problem; they were probably at the receiving end of a long line of thought about the problem of infectious diseases. Furthermore, as stressed by Walter Farber,[2] with the word *muštaḫḫizu*[3] in particular, and the Št(n)-stem of *aḫāzu* in general, the Babylonians had a clear terminology for infectious diseases. Furthermore, this letter also shows that king Zimri-Lim had a clear idea of how contagion occurred,[4] since he explicitly forbids contact with the infected woman and also the objects she touched and used.

Our sources for epidemics in Mesopotamia are quite varied as many different texts offer information on infectious diseases. Among these, naturally, the medical diagnostic and therapeutic texts are highly informative concerning symptoms, agents and ways of healing of infective disease. In addition, the apodoses of divinatory texts contain information about the general fears and hopes of Mesopotamian people concerning epidemics, and historical texts mention actual outbreaks of plague. Letters are instructive concerning specific people's views, as the cited letter of Zimri-Lim illustrates. Literary texts offer stories shaped by experiences like the well-known Erra-'epic', the story of the god of plague and war.

There is, however, another text group that is often overlooked as a source, for it is less expected to contribute to our knowledge of infectious diseases:[5] The astronomical texts in general, and the so-called "astronomical diaries" in particular. But since the field of Babylonian astronomy saw extraordinary new discoveries and insights in the last years, it might be useful to take a closer look at these texts, especially from a perspective with interests in infectious diseases.

1 ARM X 129; cf. Neufeld 1986: 53–65 and Durand 2000: 345 no. 1164.

2 Farber 2004: 122f. and 130f.

3 For the corrected reading *mu-uš-ta-aḫ-ḫi-zu* instead of the older *mu-uš-ta-aḫ-ḫi-iz*, see Durand 1984: 144 n. 97 and for a discussion of the word, see Farber 2004: 122f., who rightly stresses that the unusual formation of the Štn-participle with reduplicated middle radical could perhaps point to a ŠDtn formation, combining causative, intensive and iterative levels of meaning into one form. These combined meanings catch the idea of contagious disease in an ideal form.

4 *Pace* Biggs 1995: 1912b: "The fact that some diseases were contagious was certainly recognized [. . .], but there was obviously no perception of how (from a modern point of view) contagion occurred".

5 At least by scholars of Mesopotamian medicine. In contrast, scholars specializing in astronomical texts are well aware of the implications of these texts for medicine, see Rochberg 2011: 630.

Nils P. Heeßel, University of Marburg

 | https://doi.org/10.1515/9783112238622-006

2 Diseases and the Heavenly Bodies

It might be good to start investigating how astronomical texts can affect our view on Mesopotamian perceptions of infectious diseases with recalling that medicine and the heavenly bodies have been connected from the beginning of cuneiform culture. Sumerian and Akkadian texts state explicitly that diseases come down from the sky or from the stars;[6] a prime example is an Old Babylonian incantation against diseases:

> *sí-ka-tum i-ša-tum mi-iq-tum ša-nu-du-ú a-šu-u-um sa-ma-nu-u-um e-ep-qe-nu ša-la-at-ti-nu-um u gi-ir-gi-iš-šu-um iš-tu kakkab ša-me-e ur-du-nim*
>
> "The diseases *sikkatum, išātum, miqtum, šanudû, ašûm, sāmānum epqennu, šalattinum*, and *girgiššum* have come down from the stars of the sky."[7]

This is a well-known example of the connection between diseases and the celestial powers, which, of course, are representation of the gods, who are the causal agent of diseases harming the patients. However, this must be seen in the broader picture of the general connection between the heavens and the earth, since the heavenly bodies do not only send down diseases. By the first millennium BC, Babylonian and Assyrian scholars considered the connection of the heavens and the earth as primeval general knowledge and assumed a direct correlation of terrestrial and celestial phenomena. The so-called Babylonian Diviner's Manual is a fine example for this:

> *i-da-at* KI-*tim it-ti* AN-*e ṣa-ad-du i-na-áš-šá*
> AN-*e u* KI-*tim* TÉŠ.BI GIŠ.GIM.MA *ub-ba-lu-ni*
> *a-he-en-nu-a ul* BAR.MEŠ AN *u* KI *it-hu-zu*
> ---
> *it-tum šá ina* AN-*e lem-ne-tu*$_4$ *ina* KI-*tim lem-ne-et*
> *ša ina* KI-*tim lem-ne-tu*$_4$ *ina* AN-*e lem-ne-et*
>
> "The signs on earth just as those in the sky give us signals. Sky and earth both produce portents, though appearing separately, they are not separate (because) sky and earth are related.
> ---
> A sign that portends evil in the sky is (also) evil on earth, one that portends evil on earth is evil in the sky."[8]

The diviner's manual shows a deep connection of the heavens and the earth that goes well beyond the age-old idea of the heavenly bodies predicting developments on the earth, which is the foundation of astrology and astrological divination. It indicates a reciprocal connection of the heavens with the earth and the earth with the heavens, which cannot and should not be interpreted individually.

3 The Astronomical Diaries

Such an idea of a deep connection of the heavens and the earth is at the heart of the birth of a very specific group of texts whose interpretation has undergone a fundamental change in recent years, the so-called "astronomical diaries". This text group appears in Babylonia in the sixth century BC[9] and might go back to earlier times.[10] The texts are called "astronomical diaries" because they list celestial and other phenomena for every month of a given year; whereby the number of diaries preserved becomes increasingly dense as the end of the first millennium approaches. The diaries are written in a shorthand script, in which words are often written with a single cuneiform sign and which does not change over the centuries. They list in each month the length of the preceding month, the time intervals between the setting of

---

6 For diseases coming down from the sky, see the overview by Zomer 2021: 161–187.

7 Goetze 1955: 11 text c, lines 1–5.

8 Oppenheim 1974: 197–220, lines 38–42.

9 For a discussion of the first astrological diaries see Steele 2019: 19–52.

10 Later tradition in Ptolemy's Almagest holds it that the observation of the sky goes back to the beginning of the reign of Nabonassar (Nabû-nāṣir) in 747 BCE, see Rochberg–Halton 1991: 108–111.

sun and moon on the 1st day of the month, between the rising of sun and moon on the 15th day of the month, between the rising of sun and moon on the morning of the last visibility of the moon, as well as the dates on which the moon reaches a number of "normal stars", and the night watch, in which this happens. Furthermore, dates and descriptions of possible lunar and solar eclipses and dates and position of planets concerning stars, when first and last seen, direct or retrograde movement, stationary points and conjunctions with "normal stars" are registered. In addition, the diaries record solstices and equinoxes, the heliacal rising of Sirius, weather condition, and possible meteors or comets. But equally to the heavenly phenomena some events on earth are also noted; these include the prices in silver of six important commodities – grain, dates, *kasû*, *saḫlû*, sesame, and wool, as well as the level of the Euphrates, historical events or curiosities, mostly of divinatory interest.

An interesting aspect of the astronomical diaries is a repeated remark that the celestial phenomena were recorded but not directly observed due to bad weather, e. g. in an astronomical diary of 372BC "The 1st, the sun was surrounded by a halo; overcast. Night of the 2nd (and) the 2nd, overcast. The 2nd, equinox; I did not watch".[11] The unobserved celestial phenomena must therefore have been calculated.[12] Since the rediscovery of the goal year method, it has become clear how the movements of the moon and planets could be calculated: Babylonian scholars had discovered the fact that a planet or the moon appeared again at the same celestial position on the same day of the Babylonian calendar after a certain period of time. By calculating these periods of time for the movement if the heavenly bodies through careful and long-time observation, Babylonian scholars could predict the position of the moon or the planets for a given future year, the goal year. This enabled them to predict the time and position of not yet watched celestial phenomena. The goal year method is documented in the "goal year texts", which are attested from the 2nd century, but assumed to be used already in the 6th century BC. Knowledge of the goal year method was a basis for the creation of the astronomical diaries, which is also clear from the fact that they only record astronomical phenomena for which a goal year period was known, with the exception of halos and comets.

But why did Babylonian scholars start to write down the astronomical diaries at all, when they were already able to predict the movement of the heavenly bodies?[13] It becomes increasingly clear that the prediction of the noted *terrestrial* phenomena –the prices in silver of six important commodities, the level of the Euphrates, and historical events or curiosities were the real reason for creating the astronomical diaries and their unchanged character over time. In the words of M. Ossendrijver:

> "The listing of such terrestrial observations does hardly change throughout the time, in which the diaries were recorded (ca. 650–50 BC). Therefore, it can be adduced that the compilation of astronomical and terrestrical phenomena is intended from the start and was made concerning a certain aim. It is obvious that this aim was the recording of the correlation of terrestrial and celestial phenomena. Knowledge of such correlation would make I possible to reduce the prediction of a phenomenon on earth to the prediction of the correlating astronomical phenomenon, which was already known by the goal year method."[14]

It is important to realise what this means: by the 7th century BC at the latest, the Babylonians had understood the basic processes in the sky to such an extent that they were able to calculate the positions of the moon and planets in advance and also predict solar and lunar eclipses. The astronomical diaries were therefore not primarily recorded in order to understand the approaches in the sky, but to predict the processes on earth, i.e. crop yields, price developments, historical and divinatory events.

As evidence for his thesis, Ossendrijver can refer to a late Babylonian tablet from the library of the scholar Iqīša, who was active in Uruk around 310 BC., which deals precisely with this prediction of market prices:

11 Hunger and Sachs 1988: 108–109, col. l, 3.

12 For a detailed description of the following, see Ossendrijver 2011: 152–156.

13 According to Ossendrijver 2011: 154, one astronomical aspect of the diaries was the prediction of the visibility of the new crescent moon by predicting the corresponding lunar six-interval, which alone, however, does not explain the astronomical diaries.

14 Ossendrijver 2011: 155: "Über die ganze Periode, aus der es Tagebücher gibt (650–50 v. Chr.), hat sich diese Struktur kaum geändert. Daraus kann geschlossen werden, dass die Zusammenstellung von astronomischen und irdischen Phänomenen von Anfang an beabsichtigt war und mit einem bestimmten Zweck erfolgte. Es ist naheliegend, dass Korrelationen zwischen irdischen und astronomischen Phänomenen erfasst werden sollten. Durch die Kenntnis solcher Korrelationen würde sich die Vorhersage eines irdischen Phänomens auf die Vorhersage der damit korrelierten astronomischen Phänomene reduzieren, die bereits mit der Zieljahrmethode möglich war".

"If you want to make a prediction for the area of the grain price – broken – then you look into the orbit of the planets, and you watch the first visibility, the last visibility, the stationary position, the opposition, the passage (of stars), the dimness and brightness of planets, and the zodiacal signs, when they start rising and setting, and then you make a prediction for your year, and it will be correct."[15]

In this extraordinary passage the general principle for predicting the price of grain for the next year is dealt with and the text mentions exactly such astronomical phenomena, which correlate to the ones used in the astronomical diaries for prediction.

This new interpretation of the aim of the astronomical diaries with its shift of focus from understanding astronomical phenomena to understanding what is happening in the world, apprehending the assumed mechanisms which govern the course of time on earth, fundamentally changes our perspective on Mesopotamian scholars and their science. We are only beginning to realise what this means for many fields of late Mesopotamian scholarly endeavour.[16]

4 Epidemic Diseases in the Astronomical Diaries

Having roughly outlined the developments in the interpretation of the astronomical diaries in recent years, we turn to the question of what this means for epidemics. There is a connection between the astronomical diaries and infectious diseases, which is less known, since scholars specialising in the field of medicine look but rarely for medical evidence in astronomical texts. This connection is the fact that apart from the regular mentioning of the six important trade commodities, the level of the Euphrates, historical events or curiosities, the astronomical diaries sometimes also note down disease outbreaks.

Such notations of diseases in the land appear but rarely in the astronomical diaries,[17] a search through the published astronomical diaries yields only seven instances, here listed according to the years and months in which they appear:

-567: obv. 7: Month I: *su-alu u ri-šu-tu i-ṣa* [. . .]

"Coughing and a little *rišûtu*-disease [. . . .]"

-382: obv. 13': Month II: G]IG KA *u ri-šu-tu ina* KUR MAḪ

"[. . . .] there was much "mouth-disease" and *rišûtu*-disease in the land."

-330: obv. 4: Month VI: *ina* AN.MI NAM.ÚŠ.ME *u šib-ṭi ina* [. . .]

"during the eclipse, deaths and *šibṭu* [occurred] in [. . . .]" (in astronomical section)

-273: rev. 33' and upper edge 1: M[U] BI GIG *ek-ke-tu*$_4$ *ina ina* KUR MAḪ

"That year, there was much *ekketu*-disease in the land."

-117: obv. 8': Month VIII: ITI BI GIG ⸢x x⸣ [

"That month [there was] . . . -disease [. . . . . .]."

-105: obv 46': Month III: ITI BI *ek-ke-tú u ri-šu-*[*tú*] *ina ina* KUR GÁL-*ši*

"That month there was *ekketu*- and *rišûtu*-disease in the land."

-93: obv 11: Month IV: ITI BI GIG.MEŠ *u* ÚŠ.MEŠ *ina* KUR MAḪ.MEŠ

"That month there were many sick people and deaths in the land."

In addition, there are three further instances dealing with animal- or crop-disease:

-153: rev. 4'–5': Month V: ITI BI *di-ḫu ina* ÁB.GU$_4$.Ḫ[Á]

"That month there was *diḫu*-disease among the cattle".

-122: obv. 8': MU BI *še-im ina* BURU$_{14}$ *sa-ma-nu* DAB-*bat*

"That year *sāmānu*-disease seized the barley during harvest."

-112, rev. 12': Month IV: *di-'u ina* GU$_4$.MEŠ *ša* KUR URI[^{ki}

"*di'u*-disease [. . .] among the cattle of Babylonia . . . "

15 Hunger 1976: 95–99 no. 94, here 97; see Ossendrijver 2011: 155.

16 Heeßel 2021: 48–66.

17 Tuplin 2019: 88 n. 30. Cf. also Pirngruber (2014) for attacks of locusts noted in the diaries.

As is well known, the Babylonian terms for epidemics are quite general. The mostly used terms *mūtānū* (*mūtu+ānū*): "collective deaths, number of deaths" and *ukultu* "devouring" (of humans or animals) are not specific in epidemic diseases being the reason for these deaths. Other more specific words appear less frequently like *isiltu* "swelling", an epidemic of the land, troops, etc., *masla'tu* "infection, epidemic", from *salā'u* "to become ill, infected", *miqittu* "epidemic (of animals)", literally the "fall", and *šibṭu* "blow, epidemic, plague". While the terms *mūtānū* and *šibṭu* do appear in these instances (e. g. in the one for -330), it is salient how seldom general terms for epidemics are mentioned in the astronomical diaries. Rather, the diaries name specific diseases as having epidemic character, which hitherto few medical specialists would have classified as epidemic.

The specific disease mentioned as epidemic in the astronomical diaries are *rišûtu* "redness", *ekketu*, often interpreted as "scabies", *suālu* "cough(ing)" and *muruṣ pî* "mouth disease"[18]. *di'u/diḫu* appears as a disease of cattle, while *sāmānu*, which can also be a disease in humans and animals, is here a crop-disease. At first glance, it is surprising to find these diseases considered as epidemic, since they are not described as epidemic in therapeutic medical texts. *suālu* "cough(ing)" hardly figures as epidemic in medical therapeutic texts.[19] *ekketu* and *rišûtu* frequently appear together in these texts,[20] which illustrates their medical connection. In the 33rd tablet of the diagnostic handbook, in which diseases are described – or one might even think about the term 'defined' – in the style *murṣu šikinšu . . . šumšu* "If the nature of the disease . . . (then) . . . is its name", *rišûtu* follows *ekketu* directly.[21] The decisive descriptions of the disease are: *kīma ummedi qablīšu ilammi* "it is like an abscess and it goes round his hips" for *ekketu* and *kīma qulepti nūni zumuršu mali u adanna iraššī* and/or . . . *kīma ḫimṭi ēmma* . . . "his body is full of scales like a fish and he has (the condition) for a limited time" and/or "it (feels) hot like a burn and . . . ". Both descriptions do not exactly refer to epidemic diseases, yet, *ekketu* has been identified as scabies, which might get additional support by the references in the astrological diaries as an epidemic, since scabies is an epidemological disease. The phrase *muruṣ pî* "mouth disease" is too unspecific to be connected to a distinct medical condition. The disease *di'u/diḫu* is well attested as a disease of humans, less so as a disease of animals as it appears in the astrological diaries. *Sāmānu* as a crop disease is well attested in medical and other texts.[22]

5 Conclusion: What does this mean for the Concept of Contagious Disease in Mesopotamia?

It should have become clear that for the compilers of the astronomical diaries in first millennium Babylonia, the listed diseases were believed to be endemic. This is especially interesting, since neither *rišûtu*, *ekketu*, nor *suālu* are described as epidemic in the medical texts *stricto sensu*, i. e. the therapeutic and diagnostic texts. As for *ekketu*, this epidemic character might support its interpretation as "scabies".

Beyond the immediate interpretation of the diseases mentioned, the inclusion of epidemic outbreaks in the astronomical diaries is intriguing. The astronomical diaries are a large-scale effort (or, indeed, a centuries-spanning 'experiment') to align heaven and earth and to understand the mechanisms that rule the world. Against this backdrop, it is hardly surprising that Babylonian scholars assumed outbreaks of contagious disease to be regularly occurring and tried to explore the time intervals between outbreaks as part of this grandiose scheme to understand and predict the processes on earth.[23] We can assume that the prediction of new epidemic outbreaks would then be calculated by the movements of the heaven, especially those listed in the diaries, as is indicated by the already mentioned small late Babylo-

18 Or, indeed, *muruṣ appi "nose* disease", as the logographic writing in the astronomical diary of -382 does not allow a clear decision.

19 For *suālu*, see the latest discussion in D. Cadelli 2021: 12–13.

20 E. g. *šumma amēlu qaqqassu ekketam u rišûtam mali* "If the head of the patient is full with *ekketu* and *rišûtu*" (KAR 202 ii 3), see Heeßel 2000: 367/10.

21 SA.GIG 33 lines 10–12. See Heeßel 2000: 353 and 359.

22 AHw. 1017b, CAD S 111f. For *sāmānu* as a disease of humans, see Kinnier Wilson 1994: 111–115; Finkel 1998; Beck 2015: 33–46.

23 This, indeed, has been seen clearly by Rochberg 2011: 630: "The recording of outbreaks of disease in the Diaries may suggest an underlying assumption about the periodic recurrence of diseases that could potentially be determinable through meticulous preservation of their occurrence in dated archives".

nian tablet from the library of the scholar Iqīša, which deals precisely with such a prediction, only for market prices and not for diseases.

But what is more, the compilers of the astronomical diaries in first millennium Babylonia considered epidemic diseases on the one hand as so important as to list them among other important historical and financial data; this more than anything illustrates the importance of epidemics for ancient societies and for the life of ordinary man. On the other hand, just as the other important fields of knowledge (prices, Euphrates-level, historical and ominous events), epidemic diseases were then considered – at least in theory – to be predictable, not happening any more at unknowable whims of gods. Therefore, the effort to understand epidemics form an integral part of the grand scheme to comprehend the course of the world that becomes apparent in the astronomical diaries.

Bibliography

Beck 2015 = S. Beck, 'Sāmānu as a Human Disease', *Le Journal des Médecines Cunéiformes* 26, 33–46

Biggs 1995 = R. D. Biggs, 'Medicine, Surgery, and Public Health in Ancient Mesopotamia', in: *Civilizations of the Ancient Near East, vol 3*, ed. J. M. Sasson et al. (New York: Charles Scribner's Sons), 1911–1924

Cadelli 2021 = D. S. Cadelli, 'Symptomatologie dans Suâlam (seconde partie)', *Le Journal des Médecines Cunéiformes* 37, 9–30

Durand 1984 = J.-M. Durand, 'Trois études sur Mari', *Mari, Annales de Recherches Interdisciplinaires 3*, 127–180

Durand 2000 = J.-M. Durand, *Les documents épistolaires du palais de Mari. Tome III*, Littératures anciennes du Proche-Orient 18 (Paris: Éditions du Cerf)

Farber 2004 = W. Farber, 'How to Marry a Disease: Epidemics, Contagion, and a Magic Ritual against the "Hand of the Ghost"', in: *Magic and Rationality in Ancient Near Eastern and Graeco-Roman Medicine*, ed. H. F. J. Horstmanshoff and M. Stol, Studies in Ancient Medicine 27 (Leiden and Boston: Brill), 117–132

Finkel 1998 = I. L. Finkel: 'A Study in Scarlet: Incantations against Samana', in: *tikip santakki mala bašmu. Fs. R. Borger*, ed. St. M. Maul, Cuneiform Monographs 10 (Groningen: Styx), 71–106

Goetze 1955 = A. Goetze, 'An incantation against diseases', *Journal of Cuneiform Studies* 9, 8–18

Heeßel 2000 = N. P. Heeßel, *Babylonisch-assyrische Diagnostik*, Alter Orient und Altes Testament 43 (Münster: Ugarit-Verlag)

Heeßel 2021 = N. P. Heeßel, 'Die altorientalische Divination als antikes Wissenschaftssystem', *Berliner Theologische Zeitschrift* 38, 48–66

Hunger 1976 = H. Hunger, *Spätbabylonische Texte aus Uruk, Teil 1*, Ausgrabungen der Deutschen Forschungsgemeinschaft in Uruk-Warka 9 (Berlin: Gebr. Mann Verlag)

Hunger and Sachs 1988 = H. Hunger and A. J. Sachs, *Astronomical Diaries and Related Texts from Babylonia, Volume 1* (Vienna: Verlag der Österreichischen Akademie der Wissenschaften)

Kinnier Wilson 1994 = J. V. Kinnier Wilson, 'The *sāmānu* Disease in Babylonian Medicine', *Journal of Near Eastern Studies* 53, 111–115

Neufeld 1986 = E. Neufeld, 'The Earliest Document of a Case of Contagious Disease in Mesopotamia (Mari Tablet X 129)', *Journal of the Ancient Near Eastern Society* 18, 53–66

Oppenheim 1974 = A. L. Oppenheim, 'A Babylonian Diviner's Manual', *Journal of Near Eastern Studies* 33, 197–220

Ossendrijver 2011 = M. Ossendrijver, 'Der Himmel über Babylon. Astronomie im Alten Orient', in: *Der Himmel. Wunschbild und Selbstverständnis, Begleitband zur gleichnamigen Ausstellung*, ed. E. Seidl and Ph. Aumann (Tübingen: Eberhard Karls Universität Tübingen), 151–158

Pirngruber 2014 = R. Pirngruber, 'Plagues and Prices: Locusts', in: *Documentary Sources in Ancient Near Eastern and Greco-Roman Economic History*, ed. H. D. Baker and M. Jursa (Oxford), 163–186

Rochberg-Halton 1991 = F. Rochberg-Halton, 'Between Observation and Theory in Babylonian Astronomical Texts', *Journal of Near Eastern Studies* 50, 107–120

Rochberg 2011 = F. Rochberg, 'Observing and Describing the World through Divination and Astronomy', in: *The Oxford Handbook of Cuneiform Culture*, ed. K. Radner and E. Robson (Oxford: Oxford University Press), 618–636

Steele 2019 = J. Steele, 'The Early History of the Astronomical Diaries', in: *Keeping Watch in Babylon. The Astronomical Diaries in Context*, ed. Haubold et al., Culture and History of the Ancient Near East 100 (Leiden and Boston: Brill), 19–52

Tuplin 2019 = C. Tuplin, 'Logging History in Achaemenid, Hellenistic and Parthian Babylonia: Historical Entries in Dated Astronomical Diaries', in: *Keeping Watch in Babylon. The Astronomical Diaries in Context*, ed. Haubold et al., Culture and History of the Ancient Near East 100 (Leiden and Boston: Brill), 79–119

Zomer 2021 = E. Zomer, 'Demons and Tutelary Deities from Heaven. The Hyleme-Pattern "X Descends from Heaven" in Akkadian Incantation Literature', in: *Was vom Himmel kommt. Stoffanalytische Zugänge zu antiken Mythen aus Mesopotamien, Ägypten, Griechenland und Rom*, ed. G. Gabriel et al., Mythological Studies 4 (Berlin and Boston: De Gruyter), 161–187

JoAnn Scurlock

Gods of Plague or Friends of Man? The Curious Case of the Ancient Mesopotamian Gods Marduk and Nergal

1 Their Enchanted World

Ancient Mesopotamians lived in what Marshall Sahlins has termed the "enchanted universe" (Sahlins 2022). Everything had a spirit. At the top were the great gods, one of whom served as head of the pantheon. Beneath them were lesser divinities who served as viziers, gate openers, scribes and other attendants to the great gods. There were also demons who were sometimes in the employ of gods (as was the prosecuting attorney demon) and sometimes corruptly free-lanced to inflict illness in hopes of eliciting a handout.

Somewhat overlapping with this category were the ghosts of the dead. Some of these, as for example the male *lilû* and the female *lilītu* and *ardat lilî*, were once living persons who had died without knowing the joys of marrying and having children. These unhappy spirits preyed, vampire-like on young persons of the opposite sex who wasted away and died, swelling the numbers of these demons by position. Other ghosts could be persuaded by evil people to inflict harm, and there were beggar-ghosts who could legitimately pester the living to provide the necessary sustenance in their Netherworld prison.[1]

Further down the ladder of being were the spirits of animals, the horse, the lion and the bull all the way down to the tiniest insect.[2] Even further down were the spirits of plants, particularly those with medical uses. Scraping the bottom were what we would consider inanimate objects including buildings, weapons, clay pits, and even rocks. Any or all of these might be addressed in the course of a ritual and expected to understand, however dimly, what was being said to them.[3]

2 Our Disenchanted World

By comparison, our own world is rather thread bare. Considering the amount of terror inspired by ghosts, vampires and zombies in the modern world, it is hard for us to imagine how the ancients coped with a situation in which even rocks and trees had indwelling spirits that could be troublesome, if not outright dangerous. It is bad enough to have to worry about the possibility of one God punishing you with illness, but imagine having a myriad of gods doing the same, and not always for any discernible reason. To this must be added the propensities of ancient ghosts and demons, ever eager for a handout, to inflict illness as a form of supernatural extortion. All this would seem, on the surface of it, to heighten the natural fear of disease to almost unimaginable proportions.

But is this really the case? The amount of fear generated by something is inversely proportional to how much control you have over it. We can see this principle at work in our own modern lives. Our world is full of diseases, with even the ones that seem to have been eradicated seemingly resurrected. However, even if many people die of an illness every year, as long as there is a treatment or vaccine to give hope, there is no great panic. The CDC estimates that there were between 9.4 million and 41 million illnesses, 100,000 and 710,000 hospitalizations and 4,900 and 52,000 deaths annually between 2010 and 2022.[4] And yet I have never lost any sleep worrying about getting it. What you do worry about are the things that kill you and there is little or nothing that can be done about it. Cancer is the obvious example. Some cancers are treatable, especially if caught early. However, others are not. I have lost friends to liver and pancreatic cancer and they were gone so quickly—now *that* is something to be afraid of.

1 For more on the *lilû* class of demons, see Scurlock 2014a: 101–105, and for ghosts, see Scurlock 2006: 5–20.
2 For magic designed to engage animals, including insects, as sentient beings, see Scurlock 2022: 56–59.
3 For more on this subject, see Scurlock 2005a: 307–309.
4 This is cited from the U.S. Centers for Disease Control and Prevention <https://www.cdc.gov> under "flu" and "about" (accessed 14/01/2024).

JoAnn Scurlock, Elmhurst University

 | https://doi.org/10.1515/9783112238622-007

And then there are epidemics where lots of people are dying at once. These are particularly scary at the beginning, but scale down to a dull roar if and when the medical community gains control. Influenza was not always in the controlled category. There was a variant known to us incorrectly as Spanish Flu that seems to have erupted in Fort Riley Kansas and was generously spread by our "dough boys" to the rest of the world. Millions died worldwide and, in the US, the pandemic infected 114 million out of a population of 103 million and took the lives of some 675,000 Americans including my great aunt Tina (Fujimura 2003). Here was cause for panic. And the same may be said for COVID-19. At first, we all felt rather helpless, but once a vaccine was developed complacency began to set in, perhaps a bit too quickly.

Another curious concomitant of the COVID-19 era and beyond is a rejection on many fronts of what we would **now** consider to be science. Scientists in many, but not all, fields have slowly but surely moved away from the disenchanted world of the French mathematician Renée Descartes and his mechanical philosopher followers, a world aptly described by Niek Veldhuis as grounds for rejecting the use of the word "science" for the enchanted world of ancient Mesopotamians as having a concept of nature defined as a "predictable universe that follows an impersonal regularity" (Veldhuis 2014: 22–23).

The mechanical philosophers took inspiration from Descartes' famous dictum: "I think therefore I am" to imagine themselves as possessing immaterial God-given minds, all else being matter "entirely devoid of sentience and consciousness" (Easlea 1980: 111). This conceit led them to reject what they considered to be magic or, as they put it, "occult forces" and this, in turn, led to a rather absurd explanation for gestation, namely that, at Creation, God pre-formed all the young of whatever species were ever to exist in the womb of the first female. These fully formed, if extremely microscopic, individuals came encased one inside the other like Russian dolls. As time progressed, the little ones were shelled out in turn and got bigger without change or alteration (Easlea 1980: 146–148). Sexual intercourse apparently had nothing to do with it.

And this was not the only damage done. Every major advance in science, whether in medicine, biology or physics, has had to fight its way past this mechanical philosophy (Easlea 1980: 192–195). Indeed, the current intelligent design theory is a mathematically grounded resurgence of the view that God is life and all the rest dead matter. In a similar vein, we are witnessing the rejection of climate change and of modern methods of combatting illness. So it is high time to have a closer look at the ancient Mesopotamian alternative.

3 Enchanted Medicine

The notion that ancient Mesopotamians were literally afraid of their own shadows is predicated on the assumption that they essentially had nothing in the way of medicine, so that every serious illness had to resolve spontaneously or the patient would inevitably die. I should say nothing that **we** in our disenchanted world would consider to be medicine. They obviously had something; let us call it enchanted medicine.

Over the millennia, coping strategies were developed that not only theoretically kept hungry ghosts and demons fed and angry gods pacified and happy, but, as we shall see, provided effective relief for the majority of the medical problems they caused. And there were ritual experts who could legally help you with whatever trouble you had or imagined you were having. Not just one, but two of them with slightly differing competencies.

One of these, the *asû*, was a plant expert whose treatments (recognizable in the ancient Mesopotamian treatment series UGU, see Scurlock 2014b: 2–4) were supplemented by amulets and recitations, for the most part addressed to lower order spirits, including those of the medicines being employed. He was not, therefore, a sort of scientist in contrast to his colleague the *āšipu*, who is all too often called a magician or even sorcerer.[5]

What distinguishes the two healing professionals, as we know from the colophons on ancient texts, was that the *āšipu* was qualified by specialist training to diagnose illness and prescribe treatments (Scurlock 1999). The diagnostic system was a flexible one, allowing for both what we would consider to be "natural" and "supernatural" causes. In addition to malfunctioning body parts and specially named syndromes, the "natural" causes,[6] ancient Mesopotamians attrib-

5 Particularly egregious is Majno 1975: 40. For the imposition of the basic magic vs medicine divide on the Mesopotamian material, see Ritter 1965.

6 For details, see Scurlock and Andersen 2006: 503–505.

uted diseases to the baleful influence of gods, ghosts and demons and witchcraft. These "supernatural" causes were not part of a separate system of diagnosis and treatment but, on the contrary, behaved in exactly the same way as the "natural" causes.

The *āšipu*'s magical expertise allowed for elaborate rituals giving instructions to both illness inflictor and medicines in Akkadian, Sumerian and spirit talk (what we call *vox magicae*) accompanied by sign language for dim-witted spirits. Also included might be prayers with sacrifice to gods who were supposed to act as guarantors of the rite, making sure that the treatment worked. Nonetheless, that it was the medicine, however strongly it might need to be persuaded, and not the words or ritual actions themselves that were producing the results was well known to the ancient physician as is demonstrated in this recitation for jaundice.

> The she-goat is yellow; her kid is yellow; her shepherd is yellow; her chief herdsman is yellow. She eats yellow grass on the yellow ditch bank. She drinks yellow water from the yellow ditch. He threw a stick at her, but it did not turn her back. He threw a clod at her, but it did not raise her head. He threw at her a mixture of thyme and salt, and the bile began to dissolve like mist (Scurlock 2005a: 313).

For this reason, the *ašipu* had to hand any number of treatments, both his own and those supplied by the *asû* that required nothing but the medicine itself. So if you were a poor man you only had to pay for the medicine and, if you were worried wealth, you could have, for the same condition, a full-fledged ritual complete with animal sacrifice. Nothing said the rich man **had** to pay for the more expensive procedure. Whether he did or not was up to him.

An interesting example of the use of magic to supplement herbal medicines is the treatment for an *asakku*-demon that has attacked a stable (Cavigneaux and Al-Rawi 2002). One can imagine the stable owner, almost certainly a wealthy man, in despair at the prospect of losing his investment as the horses' dung changes color and the foals are born dead or sickly.

First order of business was to rub all of the horses in the stable with a medicinal salve.[7] That done, you were ready for the magic. The site for the ritual was prepared by putting down reed *šutukku*-huts and erecting an *urigallu*-standard. Seven reed altars were erected, one for Enki (god of wisdom), one for Utu (sun-god and god of justice), one for Asalluḫi (god of healing), one each for the personal god and goddess of the stable owner, one for Ninsun (mother of Gilgameš) and one for Šakkan her husband, the last two being patrons of the herds. There were also seven sacrifices, one for each altar, and each divinity received the god's share of his or her sacrifice: a leg, caul fat and part of the roasted meat in consideration of these divinities' attendance as guarantors of the rite. The family ghosts, whose job it was to herd away the disease-causing demons to the Netherworld, were rewarded with *kispu*-offerings.

A virgin she-goat was tied up and thrown into a pit which had been dug in front of the *šutukku*-huts. Pieces of wood laid across the entrance to this pit denied her any hope of escape. The horses were to pass over this makeshift cover in the night with a view to similarly passing the *asakku*-demon into the scapegoat. Three adult male goats representing the three watches of the night were also passed by the horses, accompanied by three types of ritual drums and appropriate fumigants. A purification with water from the holy water basin completed the rite.[8]

Whether this rite qualifies as magic or medicine depends on whether or not the plant medicines that were being employed would actually have done the job. In order to assess the effectiveness of the plants used in ancient Mesopotamian medicine, it is necessary to compare, where possible, ancient and modern uses of the same plant.

In the case of the ancient Mesopotamian plant *šūšu* which has an ironclad etymology, being almost certainly a loan word into Akkadian from Aramac, head-on comparison between the usages of *šūšu* in ancient Mesopotamian medicine with potential uses of licorice (Glycyrrhiza sp.) yielded very interesting results. Although one could not expect much from an intensely sweet plant eaten in the Netherlands as candy with sometimes less than desirable results, in fact. modern in vitro and in vivo studies confirm the effectiveness of this plant and for the conditions that it was used to treat in Ancient Mesopotamia (Scurlock 2021b). In short, the approach of ancient Mesopotamians to medicine was a "use whatever works" approach, the same orientation that inspires modern researchers investigating the plants used in traditional medicines around the world.

7 For details on the contents of this salve, see Scurlock 2022: 55.

8 For more on the magical aspects of this rite, see Scurlock 2022: 54–56.

4 Disenchanted Medicine

Western medicine has historically been caught up in a struggle between those engaged in disenchanted "scientific' or "rational" approaches and those engaged in enchanted ones, particularly folk healers known in England as "cunning folk". The rationalists served a different god, the ancient Greek philosopher-physician, Hippocrates, whom they imagined to be advocating rejecting "supernatural" (enchanted world) in favor of "natural" (disenchanted world) causes. In fact, ancient Greek philosopher-physicians were armed with an animistic view of nature in which not only humans and animals, but plants, and even the world itself had souls. This orientation to life allowed them to discern a basic truth, namely that body chemicals are in a delicate balance, whereby too much or too little of the same bio-chemicals in the mix can have equally disastrous consequences. Most commonplace is the balance of sodium and potassium in the blood stream. An excess **or** deficit of salt is a serious problem (Braunwald et al. 1987: 198–204, I–112), but so is an excess **or** deficit of potassium (Braunwald et al. 1987: 204–208, I–98).

Unfortunately, this brilliant insight was hitched to the service of a dangerously incorrect notion that what is in balance in the body are blood, bile, phlegm and an imaginarily pure substance (actually a mixture of blood and bile), namely black bile. And, apart from rebalancing humors, nothing else mattered. As a result, Hippocratic medicine, of which we shall see an example presently, had a distressing tendency to do the wrong thing, all too often with fatal results. Did they notice that patients were dying? Yes. Did this shake their faith in their method? No. So, on the subject of theory-first methodology. Hippocratic physicians and the rationalists were on the same page and with an equivalent disgust at rival practitioners of medicine.

The Hippocratic notion that illness was caused by imbalance of four essential humors in the body to be "corrected" by bleeding, purging and blistering as canonized by Galen, reigned supreme in Western medicine, and was applied relentlessly for over three millennia even though it was demonstrably killing people, for no better reason than that the theory said it should be working. No bad medicine just bad patients.

A particularly egregious example is provided by the career of Fagon, court physician to Louis XIV, who essentially murdered a good part of the royal family with his Galenic medicine, and excoriated a traditional healer who occasionally (and successfully) treated members of the royal family as a quack, the original usage of the word (de Rouvroy 1967: 151). A courageous woman who hid the future Louis XV from his doctors is the only reason that the royal family survived to the French Revolution.

5 Ancient Germ Theory

When the dam finally began to break with the advent of germ theory, the reaction of what was by now the Western tradition of medicine was predictable. The rationalists joined forces with Protestant divines to reject germ theory as the return of Babylonian demonology (Jastrow 1913). However committed to the mechanical philosophy they may be, modern scientists speak in animist terms, even if often disguised under made-up Greco-Latin words like macrophage, which literally means: "large eater". Dead matter does not "eat". So perhaps we need to heed the rationalists and to think of enchanted medicine as ancient germ theory.

Ancient Mesopotamian physicians were more careful observers and not at all prone to theory-first methodology. They were prepared to countenance attacks from without as well as disturbances within the body. Moreover, their fully enchanted world allowed them to discover, by trial and error, plants that worked then and, truth be told, work even today, and in surprisingly sophisticated ways that we are still in the process of discovering. Perhaps the most striking example of a sophisticated use of a plant medicine is an ancient Mesopotamian plant whose name survives into modern times. This is *kurkanû* which, I have argued on etymological and other grounds is to be identified with Curcuma sp. (turmeric) (Scurlock 2020a).

Modern studies have shown that this plant is rather tricky to use. The key is dosage: nothing happens with a really low dose of curcumin (the most active fraction of the plant). As the dosage is increased, the expected effect appears and rises to a maximum. After that, no further improvement is experienced until a high dose threshold is crossed, after which the plant actually reverses course and enables what it had been blocking and vice versa. This sounds like a defect, but it actually makes the plant more useful, since manipulation of the dosage allows you to take whichever tack you want or, to put it in enchanted world terms, to tell the plant what you want it to do for you.

To note is that although the proportions of the ingredients in a medical preparation are standard, the amount to be given to an individual patient as a single dose are not given in Assyrian texts apart from the odd direction to use more for a man than for a woman. Dosage information thus remained part of the oral tradition until the late Babylonian period when individual dosages begin to be recorded. This practice fully justifies the warning that the trained expert, "the one who knows", was not to show his texts to a neophyte, "the one who does not know". As with the diagnosis of illness, sophisticated treatments of the sort employed by ancient Mesopotamian physicians were not for amateurs.

6 Enchanted and Disenchanted Medicine Directly Compared

So how did this work in practice? You would think that the Ancient Greek physician would know what to do with a wound, and up to a point, they did. What to put on it had already long been discovered by the much-maligned old wives whose tales are the foundation of many a culture's medicine. However, whenever theory reared its ugly head, there was bound to be trouble. Hippocratic physicians noticed that round sores took longer to heal than square ones. Theoretically, they believed, the problem lay in the impossibility of a circle ever completely closing. The solution? You carved round ulcers square with a knife (Majno 1975: 154–156).

Ancient Mesopotamians were less knife-happy and had a secret weapon for wounds that would not heal that was unknown even to Hellenic old wives.[9] One of the uses of *kurkanû*-turmeric that is attested from ancient Mesopotamia is in salves for *samānu* (lit: "red-like"), a term that refers to reddening and other symptoms of soft-tissue inflammation and-infection.

> *kurkanû* is ground, (mixed) with oil and used as a salve for *samānu* (NIM.NIM)
> (BAM 1 ii 16).
> "Dust from the damp course of an old house" (= turmeric) is (mixed) with [oil and used as a salve] for *samānu* (BM 38583:6').

Turmeric, as we know from modern experiments, is a potent anti-bacterial as well as an anti-fungal agent (Irshad et al. 2018: 2689, 2691–2692). But this is by no means all that it does. The healing of a wound is a multi-stage process (Majno 1975: 2–6). First order of business is to fill in the hole as quickly as possible with fibrin, a cheap (from the body's perspective) and soft but tough connective tissue that is ideal for filling in spaces – like that slash in your arm. Next step is acute inflammation, which sounds awful but is the body's way of cleaning up all that is in the wound that should not be there, like spilled blood, foreign tissue and bacteria. This mess is literally eaten up by various types of white blood cells released by the body. These are visible as pus which, if white, means that the cells are sacrificing their little lives to good purpose and are winning the battle with bacteria. If the pus becomes colored or stinks this is not, as ancient Mesopotamians knew, a good sign (Scurlock and Andersen 2006: 62–66). We know that this is because the bacteria are getting the upper hand; if the Mesopotamians had microscopes and could see the bacteria, they would have agreed.

Even if all goes well and the defenders win the day, there are still processes at work that can go wrong. As soon as the cleanup is finished, the fibrin needs to be dissolved and fibroblasts and other cells need to migrate to the wound and stay there (Madhyastha et al. 2010 59). Once in place, the fibroblasts kick in by multiplying and filling the gap assisted by new blood vessels which grow into the region of repair. This complex is known as granulation tissue which, if all goes as it should, contracts, pulling the margins of the wound together in a process that ultimately results in a scar. All of this the human body manages by itself, but every once in a while something in the process goes awry and needs to be helped along. And at every step of the way curcumin (the active ingredient in turmeric) can come to the rescue.

The essential process of fibrinolysis (dissolution of the fibrin) is aided by urokinase plasminogen activator (uPA), which also promotes cell migration, proliferation and adhesion. Under normal circumstances, the fibrin is supposed to be dissolved by plasmin produced by uPA. Fibrin is connective tissue, so plasmin has the ability to loosen cells from their basement membranes and allow them to travel unimpeded to a new location (Madhyastha et al. 2010: 59–60). Not

9 What follows is a condensed version of Scurlock, 2020a: 61–68.

only that, but uPA can trigger intra-cellular signaling systems, as well as ensuring that the resulting crowd sticks to the wound and is fruitful and multiplies (Madhyastha et al. 2010: 65). But sometimes, all this does not happen.

Researchers devised a test using well-plates containing mini-wounds to see whether treatment with curcumin could persuade fibroblasts to migrate and pitch their tents where needed. And, indeed it did. The job is not, of course, done until granulation tissue has been formed and, here too, curcumin to the rescue. In vitro and in vivo experiments have confirmed its benefits for the formation of granulation tissue and the growth of blood vessels in the wound as well as the arrival of normal skin cells to help form the scar (Madhyastha et al. 2010: 65; cf. Sidhu et al. 1999: 365–367, 370–372). Last, but by no means least, curcumin stimulates the maturation and cross linking of collagen, thus accelerating the rate of wound contraction (Madhyastha et al. 2010: 65; cf. Sidhu et al. 1999: 367).

Of course, you would not wish the wound to close up over blood, disease or bacteria, so the system is designed so that closure will not begin until the pro-inflammatory cytokines released by the white blood cells have done their work. A number of these cytokines, including TNF-alpha (tumor necrosis factor-alpha) ensure this by suppressing collagen production (Yen et al. 2018: 612–613), thus preventing the wound from closing and clearing the battlefield for combat.

This is fine, but only if the inflammatory genie returns to its bottle, which it sometimes fails to do. Clever curcumin upregulates TNF-alpha at the beginning of the healing process, when it is needed for cleanup, thus ensuring victory over bacteria, and then downregulates it when collagen is needed to close up the wound (Yen et al. 2018: 612–616).

Researchers have, to my knowledge, not yet suggested how turmeric manages to

change course in midstream in this way, but there is an obvious answer to this conundrum. As we have noticed, a high dose of curcumin is pro-inflammatory, a low dose anti-inflammatory.

So, if you begin your experiment with a high dose (but not too high!), you will be upregulating TNF-alpha. However, as the process continues, the dose of curcumin will be gradually used up and, when you reach a low dose level of curcumin in the system, TNF-alpha will automatically be downregulated, more collagen will be produced, and the wound will begin to close.

7 Epidemics in Ancient Mesopotamia: Control or Panic?

All very well and good. So they were not helpless in the face of the ordinary illness, but how well did Ancient Mesopotamian physicians handle epidemics? A partial answer is to be found in a second millennium letter published in CT 29 pl. 1b the relevant section of which reads as follows:

> An epidemic (*mutānu*) in now in the city! The epidemic is not (that) of Nergal; it is (that) of [As]ari. [L]et the [tow]n cri[er] proclaim: 'Organize *gatherings* (*tapḫūrū*) for As[a]ri in the district, pray (to) the god, so that the god may rest as long as the *gatherings* (continue)' (Arbøll 2024: 17).

From this text we learn several important things. One is that there were two gods of plague and not just one. Nergal was to be expected in this context, but the other, Asari is the healing aspect of Marduk, who appears unexpectedly as not just a god of plague but someone killing people with such unceasing ferocity that all that can be done is to join forces in prayer to persuade him to rest a bit. What is more, we discover that it is not Nergal's plague but Marduk's plague that is seriously bad news requiring immediate action.

At first blush it is hard to imagine where this letter is coming from. It is well known that Marduk is the hero who defeated the forces of chaos and supervised man's creation. And, from the prayers dedicated to him, we know that this divinity was treated almost as a personal god.[10] Indeed, if you had a good relationship with him, he personally cured your ills and disarmed your enemies for you (*Ludlul* III 68–100, IV 12–17).[11]

10 Even when angry, you could approach him personally, whereas an angry Nergal was kept at arm's length. For details, see Scurlock 2014b: 650–651.

11 The Akkadian transliteration and English translation appear in the edition on widely separated pages: Annus and Lenzi 2010: 24–25/39–40, 27/42.

Moving forward a bit, in "Chaldean" Astrology, Marduk's planet of Jupiter was beneficent. So you would imagine him as a Friend of Man, not a cold-blooded killer. Nergal on the other hand, was the Netherworld lord whom only the inhabitants of Kutha had as their chief god. In "Chaldean" Astrology, Nergal's planet of Mars was maleficent. A nasty type who caused plagues, literally devouring those who died (von Weiher 1971: 85), Nergal is the god whom you imagine, like ancient Greek Ares, as chained to the walls of his temple (Pausanius 3.15.7).

And, as we shall see, you would be wrong, and on both counts. The first thing to notice that is wrong with the conventional picture is that Marduk and Nergal were brothers, either sons of Ea or of Enlil, depending on whom you asked. More disturbing is that Nergal was part of a Neo-Babylonian triad of chief divinities that included also Nergal's nephew, Nabû. This warns us that these gods, as patrons of Babylon and Elam,[12] were not invariably on opposite sides of conflicts in which one might imagine virtuous Babylonians victimized by evil Elamites. Indeed, there was a long history of alliance of the two powers against Assyria.

But the real shock comes with the ritual of *Bīt mēseri*, currently being edited by Daniel Schwemer.[13] This is a healing rite in which a man's house is cleansed of demons of disease and subsequently sealed against their re-entry. It features LUGAL.GÌR.RA, the planet Mars, as an absorbing pad for evil, but the hero of the day who is brought in specially to deal with these demons of disease, witchcraft and the like, and whose portrait is actually painted on the walls of the house, is none other than Nergal who is addressed in terms, and given jurisdiction, in ways that make it sound as if Marduk, rather than Nergal, is being invoked.[14]

Further research reveals Nergal not only as the victorious god of warfare, as one might expect, but also a divine chief justice (von Weiher 1971: 21) presiding over a court of seven judges. What is more, his Elamite equivalent, Napirisha, also a Martian, was actually king of the gods and head of the local pantheon, as we may presume was the case with Nergal at Kutha. This court, as is known from an Old Babylonian text from Susa, was a place where miscreant human beings, particularly witches, could be brought to book and punished by being ushered into a Netherworld arena of fiery punishment characterized as the "brazier of Šušinak" (Scurlock 2021a). That the judgement of Nergal was not necessarily fatal may be seen from a reference to what is clearly an infectious disease, for which recovery can be hoped for if it is "hand" of the Netherworld, but not if it is "hand" of the brazier (correcting DPS 13: 3–5, Scurlock 2014b: 103, 109).

8 Which Gods Cause Which Plagues?

So far we have Nergal crossing the line into Marduk's Friend of Man category. But he still was a god of warfare, and still should be the one to whom plagues were exclusively attributed. But was this really the case? Let us take a look at the medical corpus. An examination of the diagnostic texts reveals that Nergal and his planet Mars, Lugalgirra, the latter sometimes in consort with his twin Meslamtaea (Mercury), were indeed responsible for outbreaks of what can be interpreted as malaria.

The tertian fever pattern we would expect from malaria is clearly described in the following quote from the Diagnostic and Prognostic Handbook: "If he is sick for six days and on the seventh he gets well, on the eighth day he is sick and on the ninth he gets well, on the tenth day he gets sick and on the eleventh he gets well" (Scurlock and Andersen 2005: 36 no. 3.44). This particular reference is interested in prognostication and notes that if the patient takes a turn for the worse at this point, he is in grave danger.

Other references are specific that the cause of this illness is *ṣibit šadî* which literally means "seizure by the mountain", fairly certainly the Netherworld mountain realm of Nergal. Other references to *ṣibit šadî* indicate that it belonged to the category of *li'ibu*-fever that could be contracted in "lowlands by the river" (Scurlock and Andersen 2005: 36 no. 3.43; cf. 482 nos. 19.216–217). It also exhibits the classic malarial fever pattern: "If it falls on him for two days and then afflicts him on the third day and when it afflicts him, he continually becomes rigid, and after he continually becomes rigid, he has a trembling, his limbs continually hurt him, his hands a feet are cold and afterwards fever rides (var. flows) over him everywhere at once and sweat falls on him and then he finds relief, *ṣibit šadî* afflicts him" (Scur-

12 For Elamite devotion to Nergal, see von Weiher 1971 38–39.

13 For the Aššur version, see Schwemer 2023.

14 The text is still in the process of being edited and has not been published in full. What I present is drawn from a lecture (Schwemer 2021).

lock and Andersen 2005: 482 no. 19.218) and "[If] *li'bu ṣibit šadî* afflicts [a person] and then [it releases] him and then, on the third day, it afflicts him and pursues him, he continually has burning fever, severe *li'bu* and lots of sweat" (Scurlock and Andersen 2005: 483 no. 19.219). An inverted fever pattern was not a good sign: "If it afflicts him for two days and flows over him on the third day" (Scurlock and Andersen 2005: 483 no. 19.220). Even if you did recover, then as now, you never quite seemed to get rid of it: "It has a face; it does not have a back . . . Recitation for *ṣibit šadî*" (Scurlock and Andersen 2005: 483 no. 19.221).

The symptoms produced by Lugalgirra are described as: "If his face seems continually to be spinning (and) his head, his hands, and his feet tremble and twist" (Scurlock and Andersen 2005: 36–37 nos. 3.45–46); "If, when it comes over him, his left/right eye makes (bobbing movements similar to what) a spindle (does) when it spins (and) his right/left eye is full of blood, he continually opens (and closes) his mouth (and) he bites his tongue" (Scurlock and Andersen 2005: 37 no. 3.47); "If when it comes over him, his right hand and the [left] side of his face [. . .], he growls like a dog, he [grinds?] his teeth and his eyes jerk" (Scurlock and Andersen 2005: 37 no. 3.49), the last an almost certainly fatal case.

Malaria caused by plasmodium falciparum is much more prone than other species of the malarial parasite to result in mortality. Brain involvement often leaves its surviving victims with severe neurologic damage. Cerebral malaria produces lethargy, seizures, disorders of conjugate gaze, transient ocular bobbing, horizontal and vertical nystagmus (jerking eye movements), eye muscle paralysis, forcible closure of the mouth, teeth grinding, abnormal posturing, muscle rigidity and arching of the back (opisthotonos), and coma. Lugalgirra's symptoms, as described above are a good match for cerebral malaria (Scurlock and Andersen 2005: 36–37).

The deadly duo of Lugalgirra and Meslamtaea, known as the "Twin Gods", were also blamed for what modern doctors call disseminated intravascular coagulopathy. This produces bleeding so severe as to mimic viral hemorrhagic fevers as well as producing vascular collapse and mental status changes, including unusual posturing, as in the following passage from the Diagnostic and Prognostic Handbook:

> "If during his illness he does not raise his eyes (and) blood comes out of his eyes, his nose, his mouth, his ears and his penis all at the same time, 'hand' of the Sibitti. If he has been sick for) thirty-one days (when this happens), 'hand' of the twin gods" (Scurlock and Andersen 2005: 77 no. 3.236).

Also described are the accompanying vascular collapse: "If his arms are continually cold" (Scurlock and Andersen 2005: 77 no. 19.237), and mental status changes: "He strikes his crotch, chews on his hands (and) they have to put his hands behind him" (Scurlock and Andersen 2005: 77 no. 19.238).

Prominent among the fevers that produce this condition is Yellow Fever. This is mosquito-born, like malaria, and malaria, as we have seen, was the work of Nergal and his minions, the Twin Gods. Among more obvious references to types of malaria, these Twin Gods are described as producing a fever that is at least sometimes treatable but can present with severe bleeding, vascular collapse and mental status changes (Scurlock and Andersen 2005: 486–487 nos. 19.236–241).

There was also fever high enough to produce convulsions, but if severe vomiting did not develop, it was survivable: "If his head burns with fever and (his stomach) is continually upset, 'hand' of the Twin Gods; he will get well" (Scurlock and Andersen 2005: 487 no. 19.240). However, it could also be fatal: "If his head burns with fever (and), during the course of his fever, he continually jerks, 'hand' of the Twin Gods; he will get well. (However), if bile drips from his anus and he continually vomits blood, [he will die]" (Scurlock and Andersen 2005: 487 no. 19.241) and "[(If) the (blood vessels) of] hi[s face] have collapsed (and) his stomach is continually upset, if his illness is prolonged (and the blood vessels of) his face [are (still) collapsed, he will die]" (StBoT 36:14–16; cf. DPS Tablet 9: 37, correcting Scurlock 2014b: 70). Finally, Nergal was responsible for fever blisters, whereas Marduk only caused acne (Scurlock and Andersen 2005: 455; cf. 228 nos. 10.108–109).

To summarize so far, Nergal seems to have fully earned his bad reputation as the inflictor of deadly diseases. Marduk, by contrast, is presented in the ubiquitous Marduk-Ea formula as the healing god par excellence, if a bit lost as to how to do go about healing his patients. He was so powerful in this regard that a mere glance from him would make you belch out nasty intestinal gas (Scurlock and Andersen 2005: 117–118 no. 6.4).

But beware! If you had the temerity to play Marduk by going about wherever you pleased (without asking anyone's leave to do so), you ran the risk of being laid low by a seizure (Scurlock and Andersen 2005: 449 no. 19.77). Lordly Marduk was also strongly associated with the heart in a less than pleasant way, causing angina (Scurlock and Andersen

2005: 169 no. 8.15, 370 no. 16.17, 459 no. 19.111) and, in conjunction with pursuing ghosts, the symptoms of poisoning by cardiotoxic drugs (Scurlock and Andersen 2005: 355–356 no. 15.1–2).

As is typical of the method by which the ancient physician assigned syndromes to causal agents, Marduk comes into play, alongside other divinities, in connection to infectious diseases in which heart symptoms are prominent, but which did not originate in the heart: "If a person continually jerks in his bed, his heart(beat) is confused (and) his semen flows in his bed, the anger of Marduk and Ištar is upon that person" (Scurlock and Andersen 2005: 90 no. 4.7, 166 no. 8.1, 295 no. 13.71, 459 no. 19.112) and "If [a needling pain is firmly established] in his upper abdomen (epigastrium) (and) he is unevenly colored with yellow spots, 'hand' of Marduk (var. 'hand' of Ištar), he will die" (Scurlock and Andersen 2005: 459 no,. 19.113). The spermatorrhea and the involvement of Ištar suggest what the ancient physician called "a disease of intercourse", and the symptoms are consistent with disseminated gonococcal infection (Scurlock and Andersen 2005: 90–91, 459).

More subtle is the association of Marduk with Lamaštu's typhoid: "If one day it afflicts him, and one day it releases him (and) when his confusional state comes over him, his limbs continually hurt him, he is feverish and trembles, sweat falls upon him, and then he finds relief and continually asks for a lot of water to drink 'hand' of Lamaštu (var. Marduk)" (Scurlock and Andersen 2005: 31 no. 3.20, 298 no. 13.84, 484 no. 19.225; Scurlock 2014b: 152, 156 lines 14–15). The involvement of Marduk may relate to the relative bradycardia that occurs in 30 to 40 % of cases (Braunwald et al. 1987: 594). Sinus bradycardia usually presents with dizziness, presyncope or syncope (Braunwald et al. 1987: 918), hence the "confusional state" of the cited reference.

It is probably also the pericarditis,[15] as well as spleen involvement that can be associated with it (Scurlock and Andersen 2005: 459, 486), that enlisted our "Friend of Man" Marduk to join Ninurta, hero of the Anzû epic, Angim, and Lugale, in the infliction of what we term plague (*Yersinia pestis*). A number of examples illustrate that the symptoms of the disease called *šadānu* could easily be correlated with *Yersinia pestis*: "If the nature of the sore is that it is hard as a rock, (and) it is located either on his neck or on his armpit or on the side of his abdomen (and he has been sick] for three days, [he will die]; [it] is called [*šadānu*]" (Scurlock and Andersen 2005: 73–74 no. 3.227); "If the nature of the sore is that it is hard to the touch, he burns with fever, his spleen is very puffed up, (and) his appetite for bread and beer is diminished, its name is *šadānu*, 'touch' of [Marduk and Ninurta]" (Scurlock and Andersen 2005: 73 no. 3.225); "If the nature of the sore is that it is hard as a rock, as it grows down inside, it continually goes down inside (and) he is not able to lift his foot, to get up, to walk, (or) to stand, its name is *šadānu*, 'touch' of Marduk and [Ninurta]" (Scurlock and Andersen 2005: 73 no. 3.226; 460 no. 19.114); "*šadānu* is 'hand' of Ninurta" (Scurlock and Andersen 2005: 456 no. 19.99).

Also possibly implicating Marduk in plague is the development in some patients of disseminated intravascular coagulopathy (DIC). We may remember that Nergal could also cause DIC, but there was a significant difference. If the bleeding took place late in the fever, then Nergal's twin gods were indeed to blame. If, however, the bleeding was the presenting sign and there was heart/upper abdomen involvement, then Nergal's brother Marduk was at work.

So, as we have seen above, the Sibitti – a group of seven demons associated astrologically with the Pleiades[16] – were responsible for dramatic bleeding that developed quickly and came out of every possible orifice, surely some form of viral hemorrhagic fever (Scurlock and Andersen 2005: 76–78). As to what form, the specific mention of blood coming out of the penis and attribution to the Pleiades (Sibitti) gives us the clues that we need to identify it as an early manifestation of the hemorrhagic fever with renal syndrome (HRFS). It has been noticed that most of the cases of HRFS occur in May to June when the Pleiades set, and October to November when they rise (Braunwald et al. 1987: 729).

Similarly dramatic bleeding that came out of the eyes, ears and nose at the same time, was laid at the door of Gula, the healing goddess par excellence, but just as cantankerous as her male counterparts when it came to infectious diseases. The location of the bleeding and the propensity of the goddess for childhood diseases (Scurlock and Andersen 2005: 509–512) strongly suggests Dengue Hemorrhagic Fever (DHF).

Dengue (disease caused by an evil spirit in Kiswahili) is attested in the Hijaz and South Asia, so trade contacts with merchants trading with India and Arabia would allow for outbreaks in Mesopotamia. One of the earliest descriptions of dengue fever was penned in 1780 by Benjamin Rush describing an outbreak Philadelphia, of all places, so diseases of this sort can travel. Unlike Classic Dengue, the myalgias, arthralgias and bone pain that give it its nickname of Break-

15 This is a swelling and irritation of the thin saclike membrane surrounding the heart (pericardium).

16 For collected references to the Sibitti as the Pleiades, see Konstantopoulos 2023: 213–247.

bone Fever are rare in DHF. What is present is bleeding from the nose and mouth and today it is largely a disease that afflicts young children (Braunwald et al. 1987: 727).

Also connected with the Dengue fever complex is what is called Dengue Shock Syndrome (DSS). which is the most fatal of all and caused by our Friend of Man Marduk: "If his chest is clear but (the blood vessels of) his temple have collapsed, blood incessantly flows from his mouth (and) his heart incessantly shudders, 'hand' of Marduk; he will be worried and die" (Scurlock and Andersen 2005: 77 no. 3.237, 167 no. 8.6, 536 no. 20.28) and "If his limbs are supple, his upper abdomen (epigastrium) has a needing pain, blood incessantly flows from his mouth, his arms are continually weak, depression continually falls upon him (and) his eyes are suffused with blood, 'hand' of Marduk; he will be worried and die" (Scurlock and Andersen 2005: 77 no. 3.238, 189–190 no. 9.24, 486 no. 19.235). So much for merciful Marduk.

To sum up what we have found so far, Nergal was the god of death, and responsible for malaria. However, when it came time to assign responsibility for other rarer, but much more deadly diseases like plague and viral hemorrhagic fever, Nergal is nowhere to be found and Marduk steps forward and takes charge. Clearly, neither divinity was the slightest friendly to mankind when he was angry.

9 Marduk and Nergal in the Erra Epic

The roles of these two gods in causing plague may be further elucidated by examination of the Erra Epic. Erra, hero, if that is the word for it, of the Erra Epic, has traditionally been assumed to be identical with Nergal (Wiggermann 1999: 217–218) and with Nergal's planet Mars (Wiggermann 1999: 222–223).

Erra, according to Peter Machinist, is an Anzû analogue, a destroyer of the cosmic order created by Marduk and usurper of his city of Babylon, a sort-of anti-hero who is defeated in a battle of words with the Ninurta analogue hero Išum (Machinist 2005: 47–48). Selena Wisnom goes so far as to describe this situation as "Marduk's Defeat and Erra's Victory" (Wisnom 2020: 211–214)[17]

Putting this together, the reason you have epidemics, according to ancient Mesopotamians, is that Erra periodically dethrones poor old Marduk. With him out of the way, Erra is free to go on a rampage with only counsellor Išum to try to reign him in before everybody winds up dead.

Such is conventional wisdom. But that it is conventional does not mean that it is necessarily wisdom. Erra is not a disrupter of cosmic order, but a cog in the wheel set up by the gods after the Flood to keep the population literally down to a dull roar as the Erra Epic explicitly tells us: "When Anu had decreed the destinies of all the Sebitti / He gave them to Erra, warrior of the gods. (saying) / 'Let them march at your side! / Whenever the hubbub of settled people becomes unbearable to you, / And you want to wreak destruction, / To kill some of the black-headed people and lay low Šakkan's cattle, / These shall act as your fierce weapons, and march at your side.' (I 39–45 [Dalley 1997: 405–406). And, as the Sibitti insist, that time is now: "Do a favor for the Anunnaki who love silence. / Sleep no longer pours over the Anunnaki because of people's noise. / Cattle are trampling down the pasture land, the life of the country" (I 81–83 [Dalley 1997: 406b)

So, for ancient Mesopotamians, plague was part of the natural order. But then, when we should be giving gruesome descriptions of horrible plague deaths à la Thucydides, what we have instead is an extremely long-winded description of the social disruption that Erra produces, with everybody turning on everybody else and people destroying their own cities (IV 1–150, Dalley 1997: 412–413), so much so that it is usually supposed that the reference is to Sutean invasions, the source of the most commonly accepted date of composition (Edzard 1977: 168–169; Frahm 2010: 7).

Instead, it has been quite plausibly argued (Tadmor 2021) that we are looking at a case of malignant narcissism being stirred up by Erra. This condition does indeed lead to people destroying what is nearest and dearest to them, and it is contagious in the sense that one malignant narcissist in a leadership position can spread the pathological behavior to his followers. We know this phenomenon first hand from the recent pandemic, and, in the COVID-19 age, I believe that we are in a position to suppose that, actually, it was the epidemic itself, personified by Erra, that was imagined as producing the social disruption that is described.

17 Frahm 2010: 6–8 takes a more nuanced position, allowing for Marduk's responsibility for Erra's death and destruction.

And which plague are we talking about? A hint is given when Išum describes Erra's production of mass slaughter as "His [net] is spread out just like his capture of the evil Anzû" (III C 33, Wisnom 2020: 168),[18] all but equating Erra with Ninurta. We have seen Ninurta in epidemic mode, and working in consort with Marduk, and it is likely that the reference is to what we call the Plague.

We may remember the gatherings for communal prayer instructed in CT 29 pl. 1b quoted above. Interesting to note in this context is the fact that, in the later Middle East, outbreaks of the Plague were occasions when Jews, Christians and Muslims gathered together for communal prayers to their common god (Dols 1977: 246–252). If nothing else, this sort of gathering would have nipped any potential malignant narcissism in the bud. In Western Europe, by contrast, Jews were slaughtered for allegedly having poisoned the drinking water.

But if the plague unleashed by Erra is actually Marduk's plague and not Nergal's, is it possible that Erra was actually working for Marduk? First thing to know is that Erra does not represent Mars in the epic but instead the Fox star[19] who orchestrates his fellow stars, the Sibitti (Pleiades) (I 39–40, Cooley 2008: 180–181) in the style of a planet (as a wild sheep) (I 117, Cooley 2008: 181).[20] It is this Fox star and not Mars that is the major object of concern of the assembly of gods, since its enhanced brilliance will mean the destruction of all the people (II B iii 6'–14', Cooley 2008: 184).[21] This is the sort of plague attributed in the medical texts to Marduk, whereas references cited by Cooley to the ominous significance of an aura of Mars (Cooley 2008: 183) give the sort of ambiguous valence to be expected of a god whose plagues are dangerous but not invariably fatal.

Moreover, a careful re-examination of the Erra Epic, and a bit of help from the *Bīt mēseri* ritual, reveals a quite different relationship between Erra, Išum, Nergal and Marduk than is conventionally assumed. First *Bīt mēseri*, in which one of the attached recitations reveals that Išum is part of Nergal's family and his vizier of the street whose torch was raised to unleash Erra in the epic (Schwemer 2021).[22] Under normal circumstances, Išum was supposed to keep Erra in check as in this reproach that he delivers against Erra: "O warrior Erra, you have put the just to death, / You have put the unjust to death. / You have put to death the man who has sinned against you. / You have put to death the man who has not sinned against you" (IV 104–107, Dalley 1997: 414a). In other words, ideally, only bad people were supposed to die, which suits well Nergal's association with justice.

Unfortunately, real plagues do not work that way, and the reason they did not was that Marduk was also involved. As we learn from from *Ludlul*, Marduk's ways were unknown even to other gods (I 29–36, Annus and Lenzi 2010: 15–16, 31–32) and his punishments and rewards (unlike Nergal's) could not be held to human standards of justice (I 1–10, II 1–38, Annus and Lenzi 2010: 15, 19–20, 31, 35), although you did not tell him this to his face. In any case, when he was angry, your only recourse was to prayer (I 37–40, Annus and Lenzi 2010: 16/32) a good match for attribution to Marduk of epidemic diseases for which there was no treatment.

The action of the Erra epic takes place in summer, a time when both Marduk and Nergal went off to their "secret place" *ašar niṣirti*, their mutual nadirs as a planet,[23] which is where gods went to sleep every year and where Marduk went to renew his garments as described in the epic (I 127–128, Cooley 2008: 182).[24] It is for this reason that Mars (Nergal) and Marduk (Jupiter) approaching one another betokened an epidemic either of people or among the herds (Cooley 2008: 181–182). The binary opposition paradigm espoused by Western scholarship must see the approach of Mars to

18 *Pace* Wisnom, this is hardly ironic.

19 For the MUL.APIN references, see CAD Š/II 270 s.v. *šēlebu* mng. 2. This is also the opinion of Al-Rawi and Black 1989: 112–113 and of Frahm 2010: 8.

20 Trapped in the notion that Erra is Nergal and somehow also the Fox Constellation, Cooley misses the valence of the animal comparisons. Erra is neither a lion nor a wild sheep; he just behaves like one. To be fair, there is a great deal of confusion in cuneiform sources on this point, particularly in texts from the Western peripheries.

21 Cooley 2018: 183–184 keeps insisting that we are actually talking about Mars.

22 For more on this aspect of Išum, see George 2015.

23 Chaldean astrologers inverted the nadirs and exaltations of Jupiter vis à vis those of Mars, giving the false impression that the *ašar niṣirti*, etymologically nadir, refers instead to the exaltation. As we know from modern charts for Chaldean astrology, the nadir of Mars was in Cancer (Du'uzu). The points for Nergal/Mars are known from so-called Chaldean astrology and, as established by Johannes Koch (2006), the exaltations and nadirs of the planet Jupiter have been inverted vis a vis the exaltations and nadirs of the planet Mars by the so-called Chaldeans. In the original ancient Mesopotamian system, Marduk/Jupiter and Nergal Mars had the same exaltations and nadirs as follows: Jupiter and Mars, Nadir = Month 4 = Du'uzu = Cancer; Exaltation = Month 10 = Ṭebētu = Capricorn; Renewal Point = Month 7 = Tašrītu = Libra.

24 Cooley notes that the language associates this with the diminished effectiveness of a planet but does not connect this with the nadir.

Jupiter as an evil force counteracting a beneficent divinity (Cooley 2008: 181–182). As we have seen, both Nergal (Mars) and Marduk (Jupiter) are, in fact responsible for epidemics.

Moreover, having the two brothers "approach" one another, that is "conclude an alliance"[25] in a context of abandoning their respective constituencies was not going to be good news. Divine abandonment betokened anger, and gods' garments were washed in blood. The last time this happened, when Marduk was seriously angry, the epic tells us, was the Great Flood (I 132–134, Cooley 2008: 182–183).[26] And it is happening again at Erra's urging: "I shall rise up from my dwelling, and the control of heaven and earth will be undone. / The waters will rise and go over the land. / Bright day will turn into darkness. / A storm will rise up and cover the stars of heaven. . . . The Annunnaki will come up and trample on living beings. / Until I gird myself with weapons, who can make them go back?" (1 170–179, Dalley 1997: 408a).[27]

Marduk cannot himself act for the moment. Instead, he uses Erra to do the dirty work. We know this because Erra flattens Išum's futile attempts to hold him back by telling Išum what essentially amounts to: "You idiot, don't you know that what I am doing is in accordance with the word of Marduk?" Literally, this is: How can you speak like one who is ignorant? You advise me as if you did not know of Marduk's words to me . . . . Was Marduk's word not pleasing to you?" (III.114'–115', 128', Dalley 1997: 411b).

And Erra is by no means inventing things. In the new fragment of the second tablet of the epic, it is made crystal clear that Marduk's word that cannot be contradicted by the other divinities is for the death and destruction that Erra is unleashing on Babylonia. In lines not cited by Cooley, we have: "The word of Marduk . . . of the day . . . He said to him . . . 'Come now . . . To destroy the lands . . . Erra heard him . . . (II B 54/26–30, Al Rawi and Black 1989: 116/117). The conference of the gods follows in which the subject of concern is that the Fox Star's brilliance betokens the fact that "Because prince Marduk became angry, he decided to bring about destruction" (II B iii' 9', Cooley 2008: 184).[28] And the conference ends when Ištar points out that "Until the time is fulfilled, the [appointed time] has elapsed, the word which Marduk has spoken is like a mountain where . . .; he will not alter (it)" (II B iii' 22'–23', Al Rawi and Black 1989: 118/119). So what can Išum do? He opens the bolted door that keeps the Sibitti locked in (I 27, 96, Dalley 1997: 405b, 406b) and lights the way (I 10–11, Dalley 1997: 405a) for Erra's ravages. In the end, the extent of Išum's positive influence is to ensure that there is a remnant (V 1–14, Dalley 1997: 415a).

As we see from this interchange, Erra may have lived in Nergal's temple, but when it came time to go out, he took his marching orders (whom to attack) from Marduk. Erra does what he loves to do, but only when Marduk gives him permission to do so and only so long as that permission lasts. As Sabina Franke notes, Erra, goes unrewarded for what he does, and at the end of the day is in exactly the position he was when he started (Franke 2014: 320). In short, Erra is nothing but Marduk's minion, and his only trickery is to get Marduk angry, which it is only too easy to do. The acts of Erra against Babylon are, then, at Marduk's command and in accordance with his wishes.

Fortunately, a bit of sleep over, Marduk is ready for a more sober assessment of the damage he has caused particularly where the city of Babylon is concerned (IV 1–35, Dalley 1997: 412). Love for his favorite brings divine repentance, leading Marduk himself to lament (IV 36–44, Dalley 1997: 412–413). What has happened, then, is that Marduk has changed his mind about his city's destruction.

Išum springs to action, persuading Erra to stop, successfully this time, since Marduk's word is no longer behind the destruction as it was the other times he tried to talk Erra down. And Erra falls into line, accepting only praise as his wages for all the destruction he has caused (V 16–60, Dalley 1997: 415–416).

A bit more research into the subject, and it transpires that Marduk was imagined as a four-eyed[29] *Ušumgallu*-dragon (CAD U: 331a), a patron of witchcraft,[30] a divine midwife who killed babies by refusing to let them emerge alive (Scurlock 2014b: 593), and a Friend of Man in the sense that he let you get away with being seriously bad (Scurlock

25 See CAD Q 234a s.v. *qerēbu* mng. 3e.

26 The passage continues to I 146 (Dalley 1997: 407) describing the effects of the Flood. From there, we transition to the difficulties of finding the necessaries for the renewal of garments (I 149–162, Dalley 1997: 407–408). For more on the renewal of cult statues, see Walter and Dick 2001.

27 On these points, see Franke 2014: 320. I also concur with Franke 2014: 320–325 that the text is to be dated to Esarhaddon. I do not, however concur with her treatment of Sennacherib.

28 *Pace* Cooley, Marduk was not present at this conference.

29 The upper parts of Ištar of Durna are those of Bēl (Livingstone 1989: 19–21 no. 39). The insinuation is that he, too, has four eyes and four ears.

30 For a particularly hair-raising example among others, see Scurlock 2020b: 30–32.

2020b: 31–32). Nergal, however, delivered painful punishment. Marduk also had a tendency to lose his temper, and when he did, it was his nearest and dearest who got ground up in the ensuing mayhem, as we have seen.

10 Conclusion

In conclusion, we should not be shocked by any of this. Our binary opposition view of things is the enemy of a fully rational assessment of the world around us. Life isn't fair and, in the real world, good and evil are ambiguous categories, as anyone who has had to deal with crime and punishment can appreciate. Ancient Mesopotamians had no such blinkers. Nergal had very positive uses, but, in Mesopotamia, he was still the dread lord of the Netherworld. Conversely, Marduk was not an evil god; he was a god who did evil things because they were necessary, and could be counted on to repent of any evil that he did that was not necessary. Finally, both divinities were responsible for (potentially) fatal fevers.

Bibliography

Annus and Lenzi 2010 = A. Annus and A. Lenzi, *Ludlul Bēl Nēmeqi*, State Archives of Assyria Cuneiform Texts VII (Helsinki: Helsinki University Press)

Arbøll 2024 = T. P. Arbøll, 'Revisiting Epidemics in Cuneiform Sources: Ancient Attestations, Approaches, and Innovations', in: *Plague in Antiquity*, eds. L. Hitchcock, A. Jamieson, and C. Tully (Leuven, Paris, and Walpole: Peeters), 13–33

Braunwald et al. 1987 = E. Braunwald, K. J. Isselbacher, R. G. Petersdorf, J. D. Wilson, J. B. Martin, and A. S. Fauchi (eds.), *Harrison's Principles of Internal Medicine* [11th edition] (New York: McGraw-Hill)

Cavigneaux and Al-Rawi 2002 = A. Cavigneaux and F. Al-Rawi, 'Liturgies exorcistiques agraires', *Zeitschrift für Assyriologie* 92, 1–59

Cooley 2008 = J. L. Cooley, '"I Want to Dim the Brilliance of Šulpae": Mesopotamian Celestial Divination and The Poem of Erra and Išum', *Iraq* 70, 179–188

Dalley 1997 = S. Dalley, 'Erra and Išum', in: *Context of Scripture: Canonical Compositions from the Biblical World, Volume 1*, ed. W. H. Hallo and K. L. Younger, Jr. (Leiden: Brill), 404–416

Dolls 1977 = M. W. Dolls, *The Black Death in the Middle East* (Princeton: Princeton University Press)

Easlea 1980 = B. Easlea, *Witch-hunting, Magic & the New Philosophy: An Introduction to the Debates of the Scientific Revolution 1450–1750* (Brighton: Harvester Press)

Edzard 1977 = D. O. Edzard, 'Irra (Erra) Epos', *Reallexikon der Assyriologie. Band 5. Ia . . . –Kizzuwatna* (Berlin and New York: Walter de Gruyter), 166–170

Frahm 2010 = E. Frahm, 'Counter-texts, Commentaries, and Adaptions: Politically Motivated Responses to the Babylonian Epic of Creation in Mesopotamia, the Biblical World, and Elsewhere', *Orient* 45, 3–34

Franke 2014 = S. Franke, 'Der Zorn Marduks, Erras und Sanheribs: Zu Datierung und Funktion von "Erra und Išum"', in: *Krieg und Frieden im Alten Vorderasien. 52e Rencontre Assyriologique Internationale, Münster, 17.–21. Juli 2006*, ed. H. Neuman, R. Dittmann, S. Paulus, G. Neumann, and A. Schuster-Brandis, Alter Orient und Altes Testament 401 (Münster: Ugarit-Verlag), 315–327

Fujimura 2003 = S. F Fujimora, 'Purple Death: The Great Flu of 1918', *Perspectives in Health* 8/3, <https://www.paho.org/en/who-we-are/history-paho/purple-death-great-flu-1918> (accessed 27/01/2025)

George 2015 = 'The Gods Išum and Hendursanga: Night Watchmen and Street-lighting in Babylonia', *Journal of Near Eastern Studies* 74/1, 1–8

Irshad et al. 2018 = S. Irshad, A. Muazzam, Z. Shahid, and M. B. Dalrymple, 'Curcuma longa (Turmeric): An auspicious spice for antibacterial, phytochemical and antioxidant activities', *Pakistan Journal of Pharmaceutical Sciences* 31/6, 2689–2696.

Jastrow 1913 = M. Jastrow, 'An Assyrian Medical Tablet in the Possession of the College of Physicians', *Transactions of the College of Physicians of Philadelphia. Third series* 35, 365–400

Koch 2006 = J. Koch, 'Neues vom astralmythologischen Bericht BM 55466+', *Journal of Cuneiform Studies* 58, 123–135

Konstantopoulos 2023 = G. Konstantopoulos, *The Divine/Demonic Seven and the Place of Demons in Mesopotamia*, Ancient Magic and Divination 20 (Leiden: Brill)

Livingstone 1989 = A. Livingstone, *Court Poetry and Miscellanea*, State Archives of Assyria 3 (Helsinki: Helsinki University Press)

Machinist 2005 = P. Machinist, 'Order and Disorder: Some Mesopotamian Reflections', in: *Genesis and Regeneration: Essays on Conceptions of Origins*, ed. S. Shaked (Jerusalem: Israel Academy of Sciences and Humanities), 31–61

Madhyastha et al. 2010 = R. Madhyastha, H. Madhyastha, Y. Nakajima, S. Omura, and M. Maruyama, 'Curcumin facilitates fibrinolysis and cellular migration during wound healing by modulating urokinase plasminogen activator expression', *Pathophysiology of Haemostasis and Thrombosis* 37/2–4, 59–66

Majno 1975 = G. Majno, *The Healing Hand: Man and Wound in the Ancient World* (Cambridge: Harvard University Press)

Al-Rawi and Black 1989 = F. N. Ḫ. Al-Rawi and J. A. Black, 'The Second Tablet of "Išum and Erra"', *Iraq* 51, 111–122

de Rouvroy 1967 = L. de Rouvroy, Duc de Saint-Simon, *Historical Memoirs of the Duc de Saint-Simon, Volume 1 1691–1709* [translated by L. Norton] (London: Prion)

Ritter 1965 = E. Ritter, 'Magical Expert (= *Āšipu*) and Physician (= *Asû*): Notes on Two Complementary Professions in Babylonian Medicine', in: *Studies in Honor of Benno Landsberger on his Seventy-Fifth Birthday*, ed. H. G. Güterbock and Th. Jacobsen, Assyriological Studies 16 (Chicago: University of Chicago Press), 299–321

Sahlins 2022 = M. Sahlins, *The New Science of the Enchanted Universe: An Anthropology of Most of Humanity* (Princeton: Princeton University Press)

Schwemer 2021 = D. Schwemer, 'Magie von Zeit und Raum: Ein Haus wird von Dämonen befreit' [Paper delivered at the Ancient Near Eastern Studies at Würzburg Series, June 10]

Schwemer 2023 = D. Schwemer, 'Bīt mēseri at Aššur', *Zeitschrift für Assyriologie* 113, 51–72

Scurlock 1999 = J. A. Scurlock, 'Physician, Exorcist, Conjurer, Magician: A Tale of Two Healing Professionals', in: *Mesopotamian Magic: Textual, Historical and Interpretative Perspectives*, ed. T. Abusch and K. van der Toorn, Ancient Magic and Divination 1 (Groningen: Styx)

Scurlock 2005 = J. A. Scurlock, 'Ancient Mesopotamian Medicine', in: *A Companion to the Ancient Near East*, ed. D. C. Snell (Oxford: Blackwell Publishing), 302–315

Scurlock 2006 = J. A. Scurlock, *Magico-Medical Means of Treating Ghost-induced Illnesses in Ancient Mesopotamia*, Ancient Magic and Divination 11 (Leiden and Boston: Brill)

Scurlock 2014a = J. A. Scurlock, 'Medicine and Healing Magic', in: *Women in the Ancient Near East*, ed. M.-W. Chavalas (London: Routledge), 101–143

Scurlock 2014b = J. A. Scurlock, *Sourcebook for Ancient Mesopotamian Medicine*, Writings from the Ancient World 36 (Atlanta: Society for Biblical Literature)

Scurlock 2020a = J. A. Scurlock, 'Blind Mice and Despairing Rats: The uses of *kurkanû*-Turmeric in Ancient and Modern Medicine', *Journal des Médecines Cunéiformes* 35, 34–68

Scurlock 2020b = J. A. Scurlock, 'Just in Case: Rituals for Entering the Palace or Perversion of Justice', in: *Patients and Performative Identities: At the Intersection of the Mesopotamian Technical Disciplines and Their Clients*, ed. C. Johnson (University Park: Eisenbrauns), 23–33

Scurlock 2021a = J. A. Scurlock, 'Fixed on Death: the Susa Funerary Texts Revisited', *Orientalia* 90/1, 118–123

Scurlock 2021b = J. A. Scurlock, 'The Effectiveness of Ancient Mesopotamian Medical Practices: The Example of *šūšu*-licorice', in: *Tigris and Euphrates Rivers: Their Environment from Headwaters to Mouth*, ed. L.-A. Jawad, Aquatic Ecology Series 11 (Cham: Springer), 127–167

Scurlock 2022 = J. A. Scurlock, 'Animals in Ancient Mesopotamian Magic', in: *Magicon Zōon: Animal and Magic from Antiquity to the Middle Ages*, eds. J.-C. Coulon and K. Dosoo (Paris: Institut de récherche et d'histoire des textes), 53–70

Scurlock and Andersen 2005 = J. A. Scurlock and B. R. Andersen, *Diagnoses in Assyrian and Babylonian Medicine* (Urbana: University of Illinois Press)

Sidhu et al. 1999 = G. S. Sidhu, H. Mani, J. P. Gaddipati, A. K. Singh, P. Seth, K. K. Banaudha, G. K. Patnaik, and R. K. Maheshwari, 'Curcumin enhances wound healing in streptozotocin induced diabetic rats and genetically diabetic mice', *Wound Repair and Regeneration* 7/5, 362–374

Tadmor 2021 = E. Tadmor, 'A Wrathful and Deluded God. The Erra Epic and the Mind', [Paper delivered at the American Oriental Society 231st Meeting, March 11]

Veldhuis 2014 = N. Veldhuis, 'Intellectual History and Assyriology', *Journal of Ancient Near Eastern History* 1, 21–36

Walker and Dick 2001 = C. Walker and M. Dick, *The Induction of the Cult Image in Ancient Mesopotamia: The Mesopotamian Mīs pî Ritual*, State Archives of Assyria Literary Texts 1 (Helsinki: Helsinki University Press)

von Weiher 1971 = E. von Weiher, *Der babylonische Gott Nergal*, Alter Orient und Altes Testament 11 (Kevelaer and Neukirchen-Vluyn: Verlag Butzon & Bercker and Neukirchener Verlag)

Wiggermann 1999 = F. A. M. Wiggernann, 'Nergal A. Philologisch', in: *Reallexikon der Assyriologie und Vorderasiatischen Archäologie. Band 9 3./4. Lieferung. Nanše–^{d}NIM.NIM*, ed. D. O. Edzard (Berlin and New York: De Gruyter), 215–223

Wisnom 2020 = S. Wisnom, *Weapons of Words: Intertextual Competition in Babylonian Poetry: A Study of Anzû, Enūma elīš and Erra and Išum*, Culture and History of the Ancient Near East 106 (Leiden and Boston: Brill)

Yen et al. 2018 = Y. H. Yen, C. M. Pu, C. W. Liu, Ya-C. Chen, Yu C. Chen, C. J. Liang, J. H. Hsieh, H. F. Huang, and Y. L. Chen, 'Curcumin accelerates cutaneous wound healing via multiple biological actions: The involvement of TNF-α, MMP-9, α-SMA, and collagen', *International Wound Journal* 15, 605–617

Troels P. Arbøll

Conceptualizing a Sick World: An Outline of the Epidemic Affliction *šibṭu*

Outbreaks of communicable diseases throughout history have been known by many names, such as plagues, pestilences, or epidemics. From ancient Mesopotamia, numerous terms for such phenomena are known today, originating in especially Akkadian epistolary and scholarly cuneiform texts, primarily dated to the second and first millennia BCE (see Arbøll 2024 for an overview). Besides individual studies of this rich source material (e.g. Heeßel 2009–10; Farber 2004), it is not until recent years that epidemic afflictions in cuneiform sources have gained renewed and consistent interest from Assyriologists and researchers outside this discipline. Consequently, there is still much to learn about the epidemiological history of ancient Mesopotamia.

Terms used for widely communicable diseases in cuneiform texts can generally be classified as either specific and limited to particular times and places, or generic words widely applicable to mass death in times of crises. Though sources illustrate that outbreaks of communicable diseases occurred regularly, we often lack information about the levels of society afflicted by individual diseases, particularly how communicable such problems were believed to be,[1] and whether different social strata of society explained such events in a uniform way. One of the primary terms used in cuneiform texts for describing what researchers generally translate as "plague" or "epidemic", for lack of a better word, is *šibṭu*. However, this word has never been properly examined, and consequently, the ancient conceptualization and exact nuances of the term remain unclear.

This article explores the Akkadian term *šibṭu*. To trace references to *šibṭu*, and thereby outline its uses and meanings throughout Mesopotamian history, Section 1 will first discuss the terminology followed by an overview in Section 2 of concrete examples recording outbreaks. The following sections explore the term from a micro- to a macrocosmic perspective by tracing references relating to the individual in Section 3, the household in Section 4, the city and state in Section 5, and finally the cosmos in Section 6, as illustrated by the Poem of Erra and Išum (abbreviated PEI). Section 7 draws on verbal roots associated with *šabāṭu* in order to outline the analogical understanding of this affliction, before the penultimate Section 8 discusses how it is possible to define *šibṭu*. Finally, Section 9 offers a conclusion.

1 The Term *Šibṭu*

The word *šibṭu* is translated generally as "plague, epidemic" (CAD Š/2: 387–388) or "Schlag, Stoß, Seuche" (AHw: 1228). However, a separate entry in the CAD (Š/2: 388–389) is translated as "gale, blast of wind", though these references are mainly directed towards a disease called *šibiṭ šāri* (see below).[2] Both words are derived from the verbal root *šabāṭu* "to strike, hit", and "blow", a verb often used in relation to wind as well as designating a sweeping motion.[3] Yet as discussed

1 For contagion and contamination in the ancient world, see recently Feder 2022; for zoonoses, see Arbøll 2021b and Iommelli in this volume, as well as Wasserman 2012.

2 Only a single reference in Sargon II's letter to Aššur differs, though the concept expressed is partially similar. Line 102 describes a mountain as follows: "where the limbs of anyone who traverses it are buffeted by adverse winds" (Foster 2005: 796), *e-ti-iq i-te-e-šu i-na ši-biṭ im-ḫul-li zu-mur-šu* (Thureau-Dangin 1912: pl. 5). The *imḫullu* (lit.: "evil wind") was believed to bring disease (CAD I-J: 116–17; Jiménez 2018: 326–27), and because this concept held an inherent idea of wind, it must be related to *šibiṭ šāri*.

3 Cf. Kinnier Wilson 1956: 145. For wind in relation to disease, see e.g. Jiménez 2018.

Note: This article was written partly during a Junior Research Fellowship at the University of Oxford, Linacre College, generously funded by the Carlsberg Foundation, as well as an Assistant Professorship at the Department of Cross-Cultural and Regional Studies, University of Copenhagen, generously funded by the Edubba Foundation. I am grateful for the useful comments kindly offered by the participants at the Infecting the Ancient Mesopotamian Cosmos conference in Oxford and at the London Centre for the Ancient Near East in 2022, where I presented different versions of the paper on which this article is based.

Troels P. Arbøll, University of Copenhagen

 | https://doi.org/10.1515/9783112238622-008

in Section 8, the ancient interpretations of the term *šibṭu* in especially the first millennium BCE appear to have varied among the scholars of the time, and in modern studies researchers have proposed different readings.

The symptoms of *šibṭu* are often not described.[4] Instead, the possibly related infectious disease called "wind blasting" (*šibiṭ šāri*) might provide clues as to the effects of afflictions incorporating the verb *šabāṭu*.[5] The disease "wind blasting" produced a visible effect on the patient's skin, perhaps manifesting as one or more lesions or vesicles (*bubu'tu*) with a red rash.[6] The disease could occur in relation to the ears (Arbøll 2023: 161), eyes (Fincke 2000: 218–19), penis (Scurlock and Andersen 2005: 92), and possibly other parts of the body.[7] In the context of *šibṭu*, it is therefore possible that this related communicable sickness could refer to an effect seen on the skin. "Wind blasting" was conceptualized in relation to wind, and wind appears to have been involved in causing or spreading *šibṭu*.[8]

In cuneiform texts, *šibṭu* channeled associations with violent actions. The words "murderer" (*šaggāšu*) and "slaughter, massacre" (*šaggaštu*) are occasionally mentioned in connection to *šibṭu* (e.g. CAD Š/1: 69–71), and the title "lord of *šibṭu* and slaughter" (*bēl šibṭi u šaggašti*), is used as an epithet for the plague and war god Erra, and occasionally the related deity Nergal, the god of death.[9] Though *šibṭu* appears in connection to epidemic diseases such as *di'û*, which has been interpreted as a widespread seasonal affliction causing headaches,[10] as well as the common word for an epidemic *mūtānu*,[11] it also occurs together with words such as "warfare" (*qablu*).[12]

Attestations from the first half of the second millennium BCE are rare.[13] One of first datable attestations of *šibṭu* occurs in an unclear context in an inscription from the late Old Assyrian ruler Puzur-Sîn, who ousted a successor of Šamšī-Adad I (RIMA 1: 77–78 lines 24–25). Still, the term is infrequently attested in the second millennium BCE, and the available attestations do not increase substantially before the first millennium BCE.[14] How the word entered the Akkadian vocabulary is not entirely clear, and a similar term does not appear to exist in Amorite (Gelb 1980: 33), Ugaritic (del Olmo Lete and Sanmartín 2003: 807), or Phoenician (Krahmalkov 2000: 455). Only Aramaic preserves a similar term with a possibly derived meaning, which I will discuss in Section 8.

Who was capable of taming *šibṭu*, ensure that it did not roam freely, and undertake healing to lessen the blow when it struck? It is largely unclear which profession(s) treated *šibṭu* in the second millennium BCE, but it appears that the *āšipu*/*mašmaššu*-exorcist was the main profession concerned with providing ritual protection against plagues in the first millennium BCE. This observation is substantiated by references to rituals against *šibṭu* in the Exorcist's Manual (see Section 4; Arbøll 2024: 25; Arbøll 2021a: 245–249 with discussion and further references).

4 Wiggermann (1992: 95) discussed the possibility that *šibṭu* was a specific type of plague, whereas *mūtānu* designated a generic type.

5 A relationship between *šibṭu* "plague" and *šibiṭ šāri* has been suggested in previous studies, and other translations include "wind-epidemic" (Kinnier Wilson 1956: 144–45) and "Seuche durch den Wind" (Fincke 2000: 219).

6 Scurlock and Andersen (2005: 721 n. 100) adds that the name "may be describing a concurrent HSV2 infection . . . or simply redness and inflammation surrounding the ulcer". The attempt to correlate the ancient disease concept with modern diseases is ignored here due to the problems involved in retrospective diagnoses (Arbøll 2018: 261).

7 Scurlock and Andersen 2005: 211. The disease is occasionally listed in relation to other afflictions affecting overarching parts of the body, e.g. *ḫimiṭ ṣēti* "inflammation by sun-heat" and *riḫiṣti Adad* "devastation of Adad" (Fincke 2000: 219 and n. 1644). *Šibṭu* may have been related to fire (*išātu*) as well, see Lambert 1970: 40 line 7, which could be interpreted as "fire of *šibṭu*". Whether the opaque relationship to fever-like states indicate an overlap in symptomology is unclear.

8 E.g. PEI tablet 4 line 83 illustrates a connection between wind and *šibṭu* through the use of the verb *šabāṭu*: "He who has gone out in the world, the wind will blow him away", *šá a-na* ⌜*erṣetim*⌝ *it-ta-ṣu-u* <*i*>*-šab-*⌜*biṭ*⌝*-su šá-a-ru* (Cagni 1969: 112; Foster 2005: 905). The line after mentions the household, which illustrates the variation between individual and household followed here.

9 E.g. Roberts 1971: 16; von Weiher 1971: 68 n. 7, 86 n. 1; CAD Š/2: 388. A separate deity called "Nergal of *šibṭu*" is differentiated in a list of gods (see von Weiher 1971: 86). The terms also occur together in a Neo-Babylonian contract, see Wunsch 2003: 106–111 rev. 17.

10 Though it should be noted that the disease is not called *ša šatti*, which is otherwise a marker of seasonality.

11 For *mūtānu* as well as relevant references to *di'û*, see Arbøll 2024: 14–16.

12 See CAD Š/2: 387–388 for examples. The term *šibṭu* is also mentioned in relation to many far-reaching demons and afflictions in Sag-gig tablet VIII line 76 (Schramm unpublished: 99, 104).

13 Note that *šibtu* without the emphatic ṭ, was used as the name for a queen in Old Babylonian Mari, perhaps to be interpreted as "The Old Woman". However, its etymology was likely unrelated to *šibṭu*.

14 See CAD Š/2: 387–88. It is unclear if a Middle Babylonian recension of the Cuthean Legend mentions *šibṭu* or *šibiṭ šāri* (see Westenholz 1997: 286 side b line 11').

2 Outbreaks of *Šibṭu*

Unlike other communicable diseases in ancient Mesopotamia, almost no epistolary or administrative evidence recording concrete outbreaks of *šibṭu* exist.[15] Disregarding the generic references in royal inscriptions and literary texts discussed in the following sections, only three central allusions to the affliction exist in administrative sources from Late Babylonian Uruk. The three documents are YBC 16196, YOS 19 no. 121, and YOS 7 no. 96, and they record events where animals succumbed to *šibṭu*.[16] YBC 16196 is a simple administrative text that lists a number of animal carcasses, and the list ends: "a grand total of 44 carcasses (of sheep and goats), which died on account of *šibṭu* . . .".[17] The same applies to YOS 19 no. 121, which lists: "A total of 55 carcasses of cattle, which died on account of *šibṭu*".[18] YOS 7 no. 96 is slightly more informative, as it contains an inquiry by officials of the Eanna temple in Uruk into events that transpired after the death of some of the divine Lady of Uruk's cattle, concerning which the herdsman Nabû-mūkin-apli was responsible:

> "(Regarding) cattle of the Lady of Uruk, which graze *along*(?) the wall of Uruk under your responsibility – after *šibṭu* that broke out among them [. . .]. Why did we hear (of this), but the carcasses of cattle, which . . . you did not bring in and show them to us, and [. . .]?".[19]

Apparently, the herdsman in question had sold the carcasses of animals deceased because of *šibṭu* to various Urukeans, and he still lacked payment from a number of people. To my knowledge, these three texts are among the very few references in the entire cuneiform documentation to real-life episodes of *šibṭu*, and peculiarly all concern animals exclusively. YOS 7 no. 96 indicates that economic concerns were of primary interest, and it contains no fear of zoonotic transfer of diseases, perhaps due to the fact it was an administrative document. As I have pointed out elsewhere (Arbøll 2021b: 38), it is unclear if the text implies that the participants were aware that the disease did not spread to humans, if the receivers were even aware the cattle had died on account of *šibṭu*, or if they did not recognize the possible infectious potential.[20] Sadly, none of the records tell us anything about possible symptomology of this outbreak of *šibṭu*.

Generally, it has been shown that there was a famine due to poor harvests in Babylonia around 528–526 BCE (Kleber 2012; Tarasewicz 2017). But only one of the documents discussed here can be dated relatively close to this period, as YBC 16196 was dated to 570–569 BCE (XII *addaru*), YOS 19 no. 129 to 550–549 BCE (XI *šabāṭu*), and YOS 7 no. 96 to 530–529 BCE (IX *kislimu*).[21] Still, it cannot be ruled out that these accounts were somehow related to the famine attested slightly later, considering that famine and widespread disease often occur together or follow one another during times of crises.

---

15 Note a Neo or Late Babylonian school text containing a short excerpt from an Old Babylonian chronicle, which records the outbreak of *šibṭu* and other catastrophic events in the reign of the Old Babylonian ruler Sabium (Leichty and Walker 2004: 205–207; Waerzeggers 2015; cf. Charpin 2006: 181–182).

16 Kozuh 2014: 190–92, 279–80; see Joannès 2022: 8; San Nicolò 1954: 354. Two of the three texts were first treated in the context of contagion and zoonosis in Arbøll 2021b and then Joannès 2022. The article by Joannès did not include my observation from 2021, and it does not discuss the meaning of the term *šibṭu*. Instead it interprets the term as "épizootie", while attempting to identify a modern diagnosis, although there are no symptoms described (e.g. ibid.: 1, 4).

17 Kozuh 2014: 279–80 Text 32, YBC 16196 obv. 8–lo.e. 9: PAP.MA 44 *pag-ra-nu* $^{\text{lo.e. } 9}$ *šá ina šib-ṭu mi-*⸢*tu*⸣.

18 Joannès 2022: 8, YOS 19 no. 121 obv. 8–rev.11, only read from the copy: PAP 55 ⸢*pag-ra-nu*⸣ $^{\text{rev. } 9}$ *šá* GU$_4$.ME ^{10} *šá ina*$^{!}$ ⸢*šib-ṭu*⸣ ^{11} ⸢*mi*⸣*-i-*⸢*tu*⸣.

19 Translation according to Kozuh 2014: 190–92, though I have left *šibṭu* untranslated. Obv. 4–7 read from the copy: *um-ma* ÁB.GU$_4$.ḪI.A *šá* ^{d}GAŠAN *šá* UNUG^{ki} *šá ina* IGI-*ka it-ti* BÀD UNUG^{ki} ^{5} *i-ri-ʾ-a*$_4$ *ù ši-ib-ṭu i-na* ŠÀ-*bi ki-i* ⸢*iš-šak-nu*⸣-[*ma*(?) x b]u$^{?}$ ^{6} *mi-nam-ma ni-iš-me-e-ma pag-ra-nu šá* ÁB.GU$_4$.ḪI.A *šá* ⸢x⸣ [x x x] *nam*$^{?}$ *din*$^{?}$ ^{7} *ul taš-šá-am-ma ul tu-kal-lim-ma-an-na-a-šú ù* ⸢x⸣ [x x] ⸢x⸣.

20 As discussed by Joannès (2022: 5–7), it is unclear if the meat was considered edible, though the low price the carcasses were sold for indicates that mainly the skin was usable (cf. Arbøll 2021b: 37–39).

21 Kozuh 2014: 190–92; YOS 19 no. 129. Please note that there is a mistake in Arbøll 2021b: 38 and n. 46 concerning the month specified in YOS 7 no. 96, which was mistakenly attributed to *ulūlu* in the publication, though the transliteration clearly gives *kislimu*. Interestingly, as noted by Joannès (2022: 4), all three examples occurred in the cold months of the year. However, it is not possible to generalise in relation to *šibṭu* on account of this information.

3 The Individual

Episodes involving humans or animals affected by *šibṭu* mostly refer to groups, and to my knowledge, no specific individuals suffering from this problem can be identified in the available records. Still, there are indications that *šibṭu* was a concern on a personal level, and that individuals took measures to avoid it. An unpublished small Late Babylonian tablet in landscape format from Sippar provides instructions for making a salve designed for warding off, or perhaps treating, *di'u*-disease, *šibṭu* and *mūtānu*-epidemic.[22] Though the exact context of use is not clear from the text itself, the salve might have been intended as a prophylactic aid when walking around outside of the personal household. It portrays *šibṭu* as a concern that could be addressed on a personal level, possibly because the evil could affect people anywhere. Echoes of the individual concern for widespread suffering caused by *šibṭu* can be found in a Neo-Assyrian votive inscription on an object dedicated to Nergal, which was designed "in order to not fall ill, to be spared during *šibṭu* and carnage".[23] Furthermore, a Neo-Babylonian inscription dedicating land to the deities Ištar and Nanāya on behalf of Sîn-šarru-uṣur, a governor of Ur, warns anyone who attempts to change the boarder of the plot of land that Nergal "should not spare his life in *šibṭu* and bloody battle".[24]

A number of amulet-shaped tablets were also designed to negate various evil influences, including *šibṭu*, potentially afflicting people.[25] Whether such objects protected the individual or the household in general is not always clear.[26] In at least one *tamītu*, a personal oracle question to Šamaš, *šibṭu* was listed among various problems.[27] Additionally, the disputation poem called Palm and Vine draws on the term *šibṭu* to describe a general state of being sick, and in this case, the context dictates that it was seen as a disease.[28] In the ritual series *Šurpu*, directed towards a single individual's transgressions, *šibṭu* was listed among various large-scale misfortunes somehow related to Marduk.[29] Also the disease "wind blasting" affected individual persons (e.g. Scurlock and Andersen 2005: 92; see Section 1).

The term was also used to describe the quality of an individual person in at least one instance. In what may also be the earliest use of the word, the Old Assyrian ruler Puzur-Sîn describes the previous Amorite ruler of Assyria, Šamšī-Adad I, as "a foreign *plague*, not of the flesh of the city Assur".[30] The intended meaning in this inscription is not entirely clear, but possible it indicated that the foreigner Shamšī-Adad inflicted suffering onto the native people of Assur. The idea of *šibṭu* as something foreign causing devastation is echoed in a later Udug-ḫul incantation, which refers to "foreign *di'u*, foreign *šibṭu*, foreign disease, (and) foreign *šuruppû*-chills" in a list of evils.[31]

---

22 BM 56343 rev. 1–2: *nap-šá-al-tu*$_{4}$ ^{2} *šá di-'u šib-ṭu mu-ta-nu*; see Panayotov 2018: 214 and n. 58 with further references; the British Museum online <https://www.britishmuseum.org/collection/object/W_1882-0714-715> (accessed 07/12/2022).

23 KAH 2 no. 138: 5 (NA votive): NU GÁL-*e* GIG-*šú*: *ša šib*$^{!}$-*ṭí u ša-ga-aš-ti* : *gi-mil-lu* KAR.MEŠ-*šú* . . . (Radner 2005: 139–140; CAD Š/2: 387).

24 RIMB 2: 259 B.6.33.2001 lines 17–19: . . . ^{d}U.GUR *dan-nu dan-nu* DINGIR.MEŠ ^{18} *kaš-kaš* DINGIR.MEŠ *zi-kìr qar-du ina šib-ṭu* ^{19} *u* BAD$_{5}$.BAD$_{5}$ *la i-gam-mil nap-šat-su*. For this governor, see PNA 3/1: 1145–1146.

25 Panayotov 2018: 211–15. A few duplicates of a recipe for an amulet with stones to keep various widespread diseases away, including *šibṭu*, can be found in Schuster-Brandis 2008: 138. Note a Neo-Babylonian list of amulet stones in BAM 419, which in an unclear context on the left edge line 2 mentions: *šá* ^{na4}*šib-ṭi* . . . (see AMD 8/3: 95 ms. t). Note an additional amulet mentioning *šibṭu*, cited in CAD Š/2: 399, sub *šību* B, published by Goetze (1939: 12 no. 8), which states in obv. 14: [(x) Ḫ]UL *d*[*i*]-*'i* ⸢*šib-bi*⸣ *šib*-⸢*ṭu*⸣.

26 It is unclear to me if Panayotov (2018: 213–214 and n. 56) regards *šibṭu* as the divine weapon of Erra.

27 Lambert 2007: 36–37 line 243: *ina a-mat šib-ṭi šag-gaš-ti* ^{d}⸢*èr*⸣-*r*[*a*]. It is unclear if "Erra's slaughter" is put in apposition to *šibṭu* or listed as a separate evil. *Šibṭu* is also listed among more general terms affecting the army and the king on campaign (ibid.: 70–71).

28 Jiménez 2017: 252–53 and n. b. Line 42' states: "I bring back from the Netherworld the sick and dying", literally "plague" and "death", ms c 14: *i-ta-ri ul-tu a-ra-al-le-e ši-biṭ nam-ta-ri*. Jiménez (ibid.: 267) takes the phrase as a metonymy for "sick and dying" to make sense of the line, though *šibṭu* is not ordinarily used in this manner.

29 *Šurpu* VIII line 5: *šib-bu šib-ṭu* NAM.TAR IM NIM.GÍR *ša* ^{d}ŠID [DU$_{8}$.MEŠ-*ka* BÚR.MEŠ-*ka*], ". . ., plague, pestilence (lit.: 'fate'), wind (and) lightning of Marduk [may release you, may absolve you]" (Reiner 1958: 39). For the initial word, see also Maul 1994: 186 rev. 4'.

30 RIMA 1: 77–78 lines 24–25: . . . *ší-bi-i*[*ṭ*(?)] ^{25} *a-ḫi-tim la* UZU URU *aš-š*[*ur*] (see also lines 12–13). The idea of *šibṭu* as foreign is also expressed in Udug-ḫul, cited in n. 31 below. The word *aḫû* "strange, foreign, hostile" is often difficult to translate.

31 Geller 2016: 54 ms b$_{1}$ = CT 51 pl. 142 obv. 7–8: *di-e-um a-ḫi-a-ti ši-ib-ṭi a-ḫi-a-ti mur-ṣi a-ḫi-a-ti* ^{8} *šu-ru-up-pu-ú a-ḫi-a-ti* (see also CAD Š/2: 387). The form *a-ḫi-a-ti* is not entirely clear, though it could be a feminine plural form of *aḫû* "strange, foreigner, outsider, strange, abnormal, hostile" etc. (CAD A/1: 210–213). In this case, the feminine form may have been chosen to emphasize the seven (*sebetti*). The text also mentions male and female murderers as evil gods (ibid.; Böck 2014: 183 n. 98;), as well as "evil *miqtu*" (Geller 2016: 55; Stol 1993: 11 and n. 61).

4 The Household

Epidemic diseases in Mesopotamia often appear as generic descriptions listed in groups of three, and they occur as a sort of literary trope in scholarly contexts where it is difficult to determine if they described general or specific evils. The ailment *šibṭu*, and similar widespread plagues, occur in the Exorcist's Manual, which provides the titles of relevant works as: "To cut off the 'foot of evil' in a man's house, to make *di'û*-disease, *šibṭu*, and epidemic pass by".[32] These rituals are known from the first millennium BCE, and they were intended to protect a person's house, household, and family and to keep various evils from drawing near (e.g. Wiggermann 1992: 33–34, 94–95). Briefly outlined, a family in antiquity is often conceived "broadly, as comprising all descendants of a single male ancestor (a clan), or more narrowly, as constituting a smaller group of closer relatives" (Bodel and Olyan 2008: 2). In the case of the royal family at Ugarit, the "house" designated the entirety of a family, dead or alive (Lewis 2008: 61), and later Aramaean clans were described literally as the "house" of a common ancestor (*bīt* PN).[33] In the Mesopotamian context outlined by the scholarly literature, the household appears to have comprised all beings essential for its survival.[34]

Houses and households, including the royal court, could be protected through the use of apotropaic rituals where magical and mythical figurines were buried underneath the floors of houses. Two rituals listed in a compendium published as KAR 298, with contents reminiscent of the rituals listed in the Exorcist's Manual, were intended "to [prevent] a *š[ēdu*-demon from approachi]ng and to block (the entry of) the 'foot of evil'(?) in a man's house", and a later part may relate to the ritual known as "to make *di'û*-disease, *šibṭu*, and epidemic pass by".[35] One group of rituals listed in the compendium even kept such afflictions away from a man and his house for one year.[36] Though these rituals do not mention *šibṭu* explicitly, it is generally assumed they could have acted against such widespread evils. Keeping with the apotropaic effect for a household, some of the so-called *namburbû*-rituals, designed to avert evil omens, could be used by the Assyrian army on campaigns "to keep *di'û*, *šibṭu*, and *mūtānu*-epidemic from approaching the ho[rses] and troops of the king".[37] Both the Exorcist's Manual and KAR 298 were excavated in the house of the *āšipu*/*mašmaššu*-exorcist Kiṣir-Aššur's family library roughly dated to the 7th century BCE in ancient Assur (Arbøll 2021a: 18–25 with references to previous studies). In this house, many figurines of protective deities were excavated underneath the floors of the various rooms (ibid.: 20 n. 17 with references). Wiggermann (1992: 99–100) concluded that their looks and placement partially differ from the rituals outlined above, though they underline the general ideas expressed in such rituals.

The magical figurines used in the rituals were designed for opposing and hindering the entrance of widespread evils. They show that *šibṭu* was considered a problem regularly ravaging more than a single household, though people believed it could be avoided by warding it off magically. The affliction was therefore situated in a wider religious framework, where it could be ritually manipulated. Associated epidemic diseases could literally sweep through cities and afflict individual households as graphically illustrated through the use of the verb *šabāṭu* in a bilingual incantation from ancient Ḫuzirina: "The *di'û*-disease (and) shivers, which painfully strike (*šabāṭu*) the household, bind people in the vast land".[38] The examples presented above demonstrate that specific households were believed to be protected by such rituals. The most famous of such examples, namely the closing statements of PEI, is discussed in Section 6.

In general, widespread evils appear to have been (apotropaically) treated primarily by focusing on the house and its inhabitants as a nucleus. The individual itself was difficult to protect prior to infection, so perhaps it made better

32 KAR 44: GÌR ḪUL-*tim ina* É LÚ TAR-*is di-ḫu* : *šib-ṭa* NAM.ÚŠ.MEŠ *šu-tu-qí* . . .; Geller 2018: 299 line 20.

33 E.g. various examples discussed throughout Lipiński 2000. Note already in the Middle Babylonian period the references to e.g. *bīt-Ḫabban*, referring to a geographical area (RIMB 2: nos. 2.4.5–11).

34 The relationship between a household and its neighborhood should be subject to further examination elsewhere. The religious relationships between family and neighborhood, however, indicate that some parts of a city experienced increased association (see van der Toorn 2008: 23–24; Fleming 2008: 53–54). The household is often considered an economic unit as well.

35 Arbøll 2021a: 138–40; Wiggermann 1992: 33, 41–46, 91. KAR 298 obv. 1: ⸢*ana* ^{d}⸣A[LAD$^{?}$ NU TE-*ḫ*]*i* ⸢*ù* GÌR^{II} x ḪUL⸣ *ina* É NA ⸢KUD-*si*⸣ (collated at the Vorderasiatisches Museum in Berlin in May 2024). The dual of signs such as GÌR and ŠU was written consistently by the copyist Kiṣir-Aššur, even when a singular form was meant.

36 KAR 298 rev. 40: . . . GIG *di-ḫu di-lip-tú u* ÚŠ.MEŠ *ana* NA *u* É-*šú* MU.1.KAM NU TE-*šú*.

37 Maul 1994: 220; Caplice 1970: 118–19, pls. 3–4 *a-na di-i'-ḫu šib-ṭi* NAM.ÚŠ.MEŠ *a-na* AN[ŠE.KUR.RA] *u* ÉRIN.ḪI.A LUGAL NU TE-*e*.

38 STT 2 no. 192 obv. 14, or obv. 7 if bilingual lines are taken together as one (Schramm 2008: 96 ms. C): *di-i'-u š*[*u*]*r-pu-u šá* É *mar-ṣi-iš i-šab-bi -ṭu* ⸢UN⸣.MEŠ KUR DAGAL-*tim i-kam-mu-u*. The adverb *marṣiš*, based on the adjective "sick, diseased", can be translated "bitterly, with pain", though it directly connects the action *šabāṭu* to sickness.

sense to have an all-around approach protecting the entire household, though outbreaks of disease must have been extremely difficult to control regardless of such rituals.[39]

5 The City and State

Several inscriptions from the time of Ashurbanipal's war with his brother Šamaš-šuma-ukīn mention Babylonia, or specifically the cities Babylon, Cutha, and Sippar in the region, stricken with *šibṭu*, *di'û*-disease, epidemic (*mūtānu*), shivers (*šuruppû*), and famine (*nibrītu*).[40] Again, the generic listing of such problems makes it impossible to properly differentiate them. Furthermore, it is unclear if the cities mentioned in the inscriptions experienced all these crises, or if they were meant to cover unspecific instances of widespread disasters in times of war. It is peculiar that the limited and generic references from a specific conflict during Ashurbanipal's reign constitute some of the only historic evidence for possible cases of *šibṭu* among humans. It seems unlikely that so few episodes were identified as *šibṭu*. Perhaps the term was employed interchangeably with similar words, such as *mūtānu*, for sickness and death experienced during times of crisis before his time?

Important for this discussion is a reference in a 9th century BCE Akkadian-Aramaic bilingual inscription from Tell Fekheriye in north-eastern Syria made by a local governor (e.g. Lipiński 1994: 19–81; Dušek and Mynářová 2016: 14–19). The term occurs in a section with a curse, which warns whoever changes the inscription that "*di'û*-disease, *šibṭu*, and sleeplessness will not cease from his land".[41] The text is in many ways crucial because it provides an interpretation of these three evils into Aramaic, though that portion of the text only contains two elements in the final curse. Following the translation by Lipiński, the Aramaic text warns the land of the one who changes the inscription: "may pestilence, the rod of Nergal, not be cut off from his land".[42] The first word *mwtn* appears similar to Akkadian *mūtānu* "epidemic, plague", although it is unclear if it was a loanword (Lipiński 1994: 71; for *mūtānu*, see Arbøll 2024: 14–16). However, the second term, "the rod of Nergal" (*šbṭ* : *zy* : *nyrgl*), contains a word with the verbal root *šbṭ*, and it is currently the earliest occurrence of this word in Aramaic. Lipiński (1994: 72), and later Aramaic dictionaries (e.g. CALPo *šbṭ* with further references), regarded the word as etymologically identical to Akkadian *šibṭu*, though the Aramaic term is interpreted as "staff" or "rod" used to chastise.[43] I will return to these observations in Section 7 to elaborate on the conceptualization of *šibṭu*.

Inscriptions such as the one discussed here demonstrate that a ruler's actions were believed to affect his land, and the resulting disasters could include *šibṭu*. In general, the king's health held importance for the well-being of a country or state at large. Consequently, *šibṭu* was a concern, among many other afflictions, in relation to the Assyrian king's safety when going on a campaign.[44] Despite this focus on the well-being of the state, healers only had a limited arsenal of largescale efforts intended to quarantine the population and plead to the gods in the case of epidemics (Arbøll 2024: 24–26). Instead, healing professionals may primarily have been involved in prophylactically protecting kingdoms from a malady and/or divine anger potentially afflicting a city, country, or state, or they treated the king himself as the representative of the state when he was ill.

39 Some people who could not escape the afflicted city likely barricaded themselves inside their homes during times of plague (see Arbøll 2024: 22).

40 RINAP 5/1: 132 col. ix 7'–8', 133 col. ix 5''–6'', 158 col. viii 41'–42', 159 col. viii 73', 174 col. viii 4''''–5'''', 175 col. viii 32'''', 244–245 col iv 92–94.

41 Lipiński 1994: 36–37 lines 37–38: *di-'u šib-ṭu* [38] *di-<li>-ip-te* TA KUR-*šú* NU KUD.MEŠ. The passage clearly addresses another ruler, and not any individual. It is unclear if the Sumerogram KUD.MEŠ was meant to be a plural precative verbal form, as in other instances in the Akkadian portion of the curse.

42 Lipiński 1994: 49–50 line 23: *wmwtn* : *šbṭ* : *zy* : *nyrgl* : *'l* : *ygtzr mn* : *mth*. Dušek and Mynářová (2016: 14) translate the ending of the Aramaic portion of the text as: "And the plague, the affliction of Nergal, shall not be cut off from his land!".

43 The majority of reference support the reading "rod, staff". CALPo only lists this inscription and a single younger magic bowl as evidence for a reading "plague". Other later readings include "tribe", "spear", and "a stripe of color".

44 See the reference in a oracle question (*tamītu*) about "going on a campaign to an enemy land to defeat, pillage and plunder, for the safety of the king, (his) going and returning" in Lambert 2007: 70–71 line 13.

6 The Cosmos and the Poem of Erra and Išum (PEI)

An epidemic disease could of course also plague and upset the world, as described most vividly in PEI.[45] Here *šibṭu* plays a crucial role, as elucidated in the following. Andrew George (2013) recently provided a substantial analysis of this myth, mainly dated to the first millennium BCE,[46] and he regarded it in its entirety as a denunciation of armed conflict. The text concerns the war and plague god Erra, and it references famine and possibly epidemics. Judging from the number of copies preserved, and their geographical span, this myth was one of the most popular pieces of literature in first millennium BCE Mesopotamia (Cagni 1977: 5).

To summarize the text,[47] it begins with Erra who longs to go to war and upset the cosmic order (PEI I 1–123). When he convinces the king of the gods, Marduk, to abandon his throne in Babylon, Erra has the world at his mercy (PEI I 124–II 39). He intends to kill and destroy unhindered where he goes (PEI II Periscope C2 36'–III 27). Yet, his vanguard and companion Išum subdues Erra's violent behavior in the end, and the world survives (PEI V 1–61). The myth ends with an account of how the author Kabti-ilāni/ilī-Marduk received the epic in a dream,[48] and how various users can be kept safe by chanting and honoring the poem:

> "Then the warrior Erra spoke thus: 'In the sanctuary of the god who honors this poem, may abundance accumulate, but let the one who neglects it never smell incense. Let the king who extols my name rule the world, let the prince who discourses the praise of my valor have no rival, let the singer who chants (it) not die from *šibṭu*, but his performance be pleasing to king and prince. The scribe who masters it shall be spared in the enemy country and honored in his own land. In the sanctum of the learned, where they shall constantly invoke my name, I shall grant them understanding. The house in which this tablet is placed, though Erra be angry and the Seven be murderous, the sword of *šibṭu* shall not approach it, safety abides upon it. Let this poem stand forever, let it endure till eternity, let all lands hear it and praise my valor, let all inhabitants witness and extol my name'."[49]

The entire text served as a cultural reminder of catastrophe, and it held the inherent ability to apotropaically protect the household by physically placing it in one's home. As a result, excavators have discovered copies of the epic in the shape of amulets intended to be hung in houses (see Heeßel 2014: 59–63; Reiner 1960). Unlike other myths arguing for the existence of epidemic crises, such as Atram-ḫasīs (see Arbøll 2024: 16, 18, 25), PEI's purpose was not only to explain the existence of potential crises in a destabilized society, but also to provide a cosmic framework to deal with such chaotic forces.

---

45 Wisnom 2019: 216–244; Franke 2014; George 2013; Kvanvig 2011: 159–176; Noegel 2011; Cooley 2008; Farber 2008; Foster 2005: 880–911; Al-Rawi and Black 1989; Bottéro 1985: 221–278; Machinist and Sasson 1983; Machinist 1981; Cagni 1977; Hruška 1973; Roberts 1971; Cagni 1970; Cagni 1969; Gössmann 1955.

46 See recent discussions in Franke 2014: 320–326; George 2013: 47.

47 In the following, I will refer to Foster's translation from 2005 by providing the acronym of the text (PEI), the tablet number in roman numerals, and finally providing the line number.

48 The alleged author is mentioned explicitly in the final part of PEI (Foster 2005: 910), and he was attributed with its authorship in later Mesopotamian scholarship as well. In a Late Babylonian list from Uruk of Mesopotamian kings and their primary scholars (*ummânu*), one Kabti-ilāni/ilī-Marduk is described as the scholar of [Ibb]i-Sîn, the last Sumerian king of the Ur III period (van Dijk 1962: 44–45). However, Helle (2018: 233) recently suggested that the remains of a single vertical wedge of a sign directly before the divine name Sîn on a photograph of the tablet, otherwise kept in Iraq, can be tentatively read as: [$^{\text{d?}}$*na*$^{?}$-*ra*]*m*$^{?}$-^{d}30. Though it must still be considered a preliminary reconstruction, Helle considers Naram-Sîn a more suitable reconstruction, because the king is listed directly after Gilgamesh – both kings regarded as authors of *narû*-literature – and the copyists of stories regarding Naram-Sîn also dedicated authorship of the Cuthean Legend to the god Erra (ibid.). I add here that Erra may have played an even greater role for Naram-Sîn during his reign, as suggested by the Old Babylonian stories revolving around this king, although only the associated deity Nergal played a role during Naram-Sîn's reign, as he is described as "caretaker" in the Bāṣetkī inscription (see Wiggermann 1999: 217). Nonetheless, the city Kish was central to the Old Akkadian kings, as the place from where Sargon established the dynasty, and Steinkeller (2004: 175–176) has shown that the reading KIŠ^{ra} in certain third millennium personal names could be read as *erra*$_{\text{x}}$.

49 Translation according to Foster 2005: 910–911, with only the two words for plague replaced by the original Akkadian; Cagni 1969: 126–129 tablet V lines 48–61: *u ki-a-am iq-ta-bi qu-ra-du* ^{d}*èr-ra* [49] DINGIR *šá za-ma-ru šá-a-šú i-na-du ina a-šìr-ti-šú lik-tam-me-ra ḫé-gál-lum* [50] *ù šá ú-šam-sa-ku a-a iṣ-ṣi-na qut-rin-na* [51] LUGAL *šá šu-mi ú-šar-bu-ú li-be-el kib-ra-a-ti* [52] NUN *šá ta-nit-ti qar-ra-du-ti-ia i-dab-bu-bu ma-ḫi-ra a-a ir-ši* [53] ^{lú}NAR *šá i-ṣar-ra-ḫu ul i-mat ina šip/šib-ṭi* [54] UGU ⌜LUGAL *u* NUN⌝ *da-mì-iq at-mu-šú* [55] ^{lú}A.BA *šá iḫ-ḫa-zu i-šet ina* KUR ^{lú}KÚR *i-kab-bit ina* KUR-*šú* [56] *ina a-šìr-ti um-ma-a-ni a-šar ka-a-an šu-mì i-zak-ka-ru ú-zu-un-šú-nu a-pet-ti* [57] *ina* É *a-šar ṭup-pu šá-a-šú šak-nu* ^{d}*èr-ra li-gug-ma liš-gi-šú* ^{d}*si-bi-it-t[i]* [58] *pa-tar šip/šib-ṭi ul i-ṭe-ḫi-šu-ma šá-lim-tu šak-na-as-su* [59] *za-ma-ru šá-a-šú a-na ma-ti-ma liš-šá-kin-ma li-kun ga-du ul-la* [60] *ma-ta-a-ti nap-ḫar-ši-na liš-ma-ma li-na-da qur-di-ia* [61] UN.MEŠ *da-ád-me li-mu-ra-ma li-šar-ba-a šu-mì.*

As argued by Machinist (1981: 403), the epic related the disorderly Erra to an aspect of the orderly Marduk (see also Noegel 2011: 190). Through this association, the epic created an antithesis to the arranged cosmos, which could be managed and understood. For example, it describes vividly how the actions of Erra caused demons to run loose (Foster 2005: 889 lines 175–178, 869 Periscope C2 71'). Such disease-causing evils may therefore have been situated within the regular system of first millennium Mesopotamian medical beliefs, though the reason for these demons running wild was inherently different in PEI. This framework explains how disease caused by epidemic outbreaks, albeit situated in connection to war and strife in PEI, was able to spread throughout society at large.

Besides PEI's clear relationship to *āšipūtu*, it also provided an astronomical framework, which situated the myth in the scholarly context of the astrologer (*ṭupšar Enūma Anu Enlil*; see Noegel 2011). Erra could be conceptualized as the ill portending planet Mars, the planet ordinarily associated with Nergal (Koch-Westenholz 1995: 128–129), and it was also referred to as *Ṣalbatānu* and called the "star of *šibṭu* (and) *mūtānu*" (CAD Š/2: 387). However, it was not only Mars that could foreshadow *šibṭu*. An eclipse of the sun, representing Šamaš, could foreshadow the death of the ruler and an outbreak of plague.[50] Such omens might hint at the fact that the fate of the ruler was tied to the state, which could accordingly be stricken by a deadly fate. Though the epic and its extracts were meant to protect households, their effect during outbreaks of epidemics must have been limited. Nonetheless, PEI's condemnation of war served as a cultural reminder (George 2013: 48), which in turn made sure people did not forget the existence of associated afflictions, such as widespread illness.[51] However, the individual amulets protected households and individuals, not the city or kingdom at large.

Erra was a deity attested since the 3rd millennium BCE, he was closely related to Nergal, the god of death (von Weiher 1971: 83–87), and Erra has been interpreted as a god of war (George 2013: 47, 56, 62), of destruction (Cagni 1969: 237–238 and 259; see Lambert 1973: 356; Cagni 1977: 15–16), of scorched earth (Roberts 1971: 16), of plague (von Weiher 1971: 85; see discussion in Hruška 1973: 3 n. 2), and even as a deity of death (Wiggermann 1999: 17). Numerous interpretations of Erra's name have been proposed (see Wiggermann 1999: 217–218), and Roberts (1971: 13) suggested that the name was derived from the Semitic root **ḫ-r-r* "to scorch, char", though this possible conceptualization of the god would have occurred before the root entered into Akkadian as *erēru(m)* "to be dry" or D-stem "to desiccate, dry out".[52] Alternatively, Steinkeller (2004: 176 n. 7) has discussed the possibility that Erra etymologically could be derived from Sumerian /er-a/ or /ir-a/ "strong", though he admits this development may be unlikely. It is noteworthy that Erra's name could originally be written with the sign KIŠ or the sign GÌR, the latter of which can be read *patru* "dagger, sword" in Akkadian, possibly similar to the phrase "sword of *šibṭu*" in the final section of PEI (see above).

The god Erra had a specific relationship to *šibṭu* on account of the ending of PEI quoted above, though this connection can also be observed outside this context.[53] The references to *šibṭu* in PEI, however, are relatively few, and they can even be subject to interpretation. Besides the final section mentioning the "sword of *šibṭu*", two signs which can be read as *šibṭu*, though often interpreted as *šipṭu* "judgement, punishment", occur in only four passages: (1) "I (Marduk) rose from my seat and the government (*ši-piṭ*) of heaven and earth dissolved";[54] (2) "for that time I (Erra) will govern and keep strong the regulation (*ši-piṭ*) of heaven and earth";[55] (3) "he who did not die in battle will die in the epidemic (*šib-ṭi*), he who did not die in the epidemic (*šib-ṭi*), the enemy will plunder him";[56] and (4) "let the singer who chants it

---

50 "If the sun is eclipsed in Nisannu there will be an outbreak of *šibṭu* in the country, the king will die" (CAD/2: 387 2'). See also e.g. Al-Rawi and George 1991–92: 68.

51 It might be difficult to imagine how people could forget the existence of widespread disease, but even today, before the spread of COVID-19, few considered a worldwide pandemic a potential reality affecting their everyday life.

52 E.g. Köcher 1965. Note that CAD E: 280 lists the root *erēru* as "to be moldy". Note also the critique of Robert's proposed etymology by Nakata 1979: 63–64.

53 For example, a bilingual incantation referencing widespread evils, such as *šibṭu*, refers directly to Erra in the sentence: "Great Erra who strikes people down in the street, who does not leave the small (or) the great behind him", STT 2 no. 192 obv. 10 (or 5 if the bilingual lines are counted as one) [d]*èr-ra ra-ba-a šá ina* ⸢*su*⸣*-qí ni-ši ú-šam-qa-tú ṣe-eḫ-*⸢*ra*?⸣ *ra-ba-a ana ar-ki-šú la iz-zi-bu* (cf. obv. 14 quoted above, Schramm 2008: 95–96 ms. C).

54 Cagni 1969: 72 I 133: *ina šub-*[*t*]*i-ia at-bi-ma ši-piṭ* AN-*e u* KI-*tim up-ta-aṭ-ṭir*. Translation according to Noegel (2011: 175); see Foster (2005: 887): "When I left my dwelling, the regulation of heaven and earth disintegrated".

55 Cagni 1969: 78 I 182: *a-di ul-la a-rad-di-ma ši-piṭ* AN-*e u* KI-*tim ú-dan-na-an*. Translation according to Foster (2005: 890); see Noegel 2011: 175. The translation "regulation" does not occur in CAD Š/3: 91–93 or in AHw: 1247.

56 Cagni 1969: 112 IV 76–77: *šá ina q*[*ab*]*-lu* ⸢*la*⸣ [*i*]*m-tu-tu i-mat ina šip-ṭi* [77] *šá ina šip-ṭi* ⸢*la*⸣ *im-*⸢*tu*⸣*-tu i-*⸢*šal*⸣*-lal-šú* [lú]NAR. Translation according to Foster (2005: 905); see Noegel 2011: 179.

not die from pestilence (*ina šib-ṭi*)".[57] Incidentally, these examples all inherently invoke the word *šibṭu* to the reader, though not necessarily the ideal reading in every line, and this ambiguity situates *šibṭu* as a theme closely connected to the concept of *šipṭu* in PEI.[58] I will explore this relationship further in Section 7.

Erra's rampage, mirroring the onslaught of war, must have provided a potent metaphor for the lived experience of suffering famine and spread of infectious diseases, analogically representing the effects of war. Though some rituals attempted to appease individual diseases by providing substitutes of animal blood or flesh, which the demons presumably consumed, there was no substitute for Erra's ferocious rage, thus resulting in him feeding directly on humans.[59] The universe is afflicted in PEI, hence there was no need for interpretations of contamination; it was self-explanatory that the onslaught in question overcame everyone. It cannot be ignored that the onslaught of an epidemic disease might have been envisioned as a devastating flood, as a Late Babylonian commentary interprets an epidemic as "a waterless flood".[60] In connection to this idea, providing a conceptual – albeit hermeneutical – link between water and widespread and severe disease, it is noticeably that the Sumerian King List provides the description a-ma-ru ba-ùr, "The Flood swept thereover" (Jacobsen 1939: 76–77 and n. 35). The verb ùr could be read *šabāṭu* in Akkadian, which supports the image of a widespread and severe disease sweeping over the entirety of a country as the all-destroying Flood. However, PEI contains one major paradox. Why does a text designed to physically keep epidemic afflictions away make practically no references to epidemics?

7 The Verbal Root Behind *Šibṭu*

The writing *šibṭu*/*šipṭu* occur in at least five passages throughout the five tablets of the text, though various translators have struggled with this duality and accordingly translated the instances differently.[61] This is primarily because the initial cuneiform sign in these words, namely the sign ME, can represent both the phonetic values *šib* and *šip* followed by the sign for *ṭu* or *ṭi*. Focusing on the word *šipṭu*, there are two related words attested, namely one meaning "judgement, verdict, punishment, threat" and the related term "ruling, strict order, reprimand" (see CAD Š/3: 91–93). These are both derived from the two connected verbal roots *šapāṭu* (*i*/*i*) "to issue orders, give judgement, exercise authority" and *šapāṭu* (*a*/*u*) "to inform (strictly), reprimand" (AHw: 1172; CAD Š/1: 450–451; CDA: 357). As demonstrated by the dictionaries, both these verbs had different vocalization originally, they were mainly active in the Old Babylonian period (particularly in Mari), and they largely appear to have fallen out of use by the first millennium BCE. Considering the meanings "judgement" and "punishment", the semantic range covered by the noun *šipṭu* overlap with *šibṭu*, in the sense that a catastrophic outbreak of sickness could have been envisioned as a judgement or a divine punishment. On account of these overlaps, the CAD (Š/3: 92) therefore stated that it is unclear whether *šibṭu* and *šipṭu* were pronounced similarly in the early first millennium BCE.

There is further evidence to speak in favor of an overlap between these homonymous words. There exists a rare word for staff, *šabbiṭu*, which was derived from the motion denoted by the verbal root *šabāṭu* "to strike, hit, blow, sweep", and it was used to refer to the scepter of the god Nergal in the Underworld Vision of a Neo-Assyrian Prince.[62]

57 Cagni 1969: 128 V 53: [lú]NAR *šá i-ṣar-ra-ḫu ul i-mat ina šip-ṭi*. Translation according to Foster (2005: 911); see Noegel (2011: 181) who also suggested that this phrase could be understood as a reference to *šiptu* "incantation".

58 Though the idea that ambiguous readings or wordplay should occur in this serious text may seem strange, the author(s) used these as literary devices meant to engage the reader in the scholarship inherent in the work (see Noegel 2011: 190). For *šipṭu*/*šibṭu* in PEI, see also Edzard 1976–80: 169.

59 Epidemics as devouring by gods is discussed in depth in Attia's contribution to this volume, where she provides a brilliant analysis of the visual and physical reality behind this disease concept.

60 BM 47447 obv. 4: . . . *a-bu-bu la* A.MEŠ : *mu-ta-nu*; see Arbøll 2024: 16 and n. 23.

61 E.g. Noegel (2011: 181–182) "destruction" and "plague"; (Foster 2005: 911) "pestilence"; Machinist and Sasson (1983: 224–225) "governing order" and "destruction, punishment"; Roberts (1971: 16) "affray, massacre"; Cagni (1977: 60) "destruction".

62 See CAD Š/1: 10; SAA 3 no. 32 rev. 15: *[ri-g]im-šu ú-dan-nin-am-ma ki-ma* UD-*me š[e-g]i-i ez-zi-iš e-li-ia i-šá-as-si šab-bi-ṭu si-mat* DINGIR-*ti-šú šá ki-ma ba-áš-me pu-luḫ-tu ma-lu-ú*, "He (Nergal) raised his voice, crying out like a howling storm in fury against me and drawing toward me the sceptre, which is so fitting to his godhead, and which is as dreadful as a viper, to kill me", translation follows SAA 3. Otherwise, the main references are derived from Gilgamesh tablet XII lines 19 and 39 (George 2003: 728–729). In select instances, [giš]MA.NU in Sumerian – a generic word for a ruler's staff –could be read *šabbiṭu* in Akkadian (Bramanti 2017: 125). All examples therefore originate in learned texts from the

As noted in Section 5, a word spelled *šbṭ* was also employed in an Aramaic inscription from Tell Fekheriye to describe the rod of Nergal in an Aramaic rendition of the Akkadian inscription, which contained the word *šibṭu*. And in several inscriptions of Aššurnaṣirpal II, the Sumerogram GIDRU, meaning "staff" and ordinarily read *ḫaṭṭu*, was used in contexts where it is clear that "judgement" was meant.[63] Akkadian *šibṭu* and *šipṭu* therefore seems to have held some inherent relationship to the idea of a (divine) ruler's rod. This rod, in turn, was likely conceptualized as a (divine) powerful stick-like tool wielded by kings, gods, and viziers from the 3rd millennium BCE onwards (Bramanti 2017: 134–138; see Ambos and Krauskopf 2010: 129). Considering the relationship between contemporary words in the Neo-Assyrian period derived from the verbal root *š-b-ṭ* in both Akkadian and Aramaic, the evidence points to an amalgam of meanings, and possibly pronunciations, between *šibṭu* and *šipṭu*.

Returning to the passages in PEI, I propose that several instances where these word appear were vague on purpose, and it is not certain that one or the other meaning was meant exclusively. The ancient editors of PEI may even have enjoyed the complementing meanings. In several instances in the epic, the writing refers to a crisis, though we cannot know for certain if this was due to sickness.

8 What was *Šibṭu*?

How did the ancient Assyrians and Babylonians conceptualize *šibṭu*? As discussed by Walter Scheidel (2017: 291–342 especially 331), the spread of plagues in pre-modern agrarian societies coincided with stagnation of living standards due to climate shifts, poor harvests, reduction of livestock, and famine. PEI encapsulated similar ideas in a single catastrophic event related to war, violence, famine, and epidemic disease (see also Taylor 2017: 88–99). Famine, for example, often leads to the spread of contagious diseases. Accordingly, it cannot be concluded that *šibṭu* in Assyria and Babylonia during the 1st millennium BCE referred exclusively to an epidemic sickness, at least from a modern perspective.

The term *šibṭu* incorporated nuanced meanings relating to battle and mindless slaughter, though it was also used as a term for fatal infectious disease in a few specific examples. Furthermore, it was likely related to the idea of a divine rod for beating as well as notions of judgement and punishment. In my opinion, *the term encapsulated a devastating blow towards an individual, such as a ruler, or society at large, causing sickness and poor states of health, and possibly administered as a punishment by a deity through a rod.* In its conceptualization, it may not have differed much from descriptions of diseases caused by a deity "hitting" (*maḫāṣu*) or "attacking" (*maqātu*) a patient (see Salin 2015). In PEI, *šibṭu* appears to have had a divine cause, though it is difficult to properly differentiate it from the other horrors of war and violence experienced by a community in such times of crisis.

How should we translate a generic term encapsulating devastating divine blows towards all aspects of society? Cagni (1977: 60), who published the primary text edition of PEI, translated the word as "destruction", whereas other suggestions include "affray" or "massacre" (e.g. Roberts 1971: 16). But the majority of translators continue to prefer the interpretation "epidemic" or "plague". For the present, it remains necessary to translate the term according to context, though the nuances of the word go beyond epidemic disease, and it must be emphasized that some instances may not necessarily have been directly caused by sickness alone.

9 Conclusion

Previous literature has regarded *šibṭu* as a general term used to designate occurrences of infectious and widespread disease in ancient Mesopotamia, most frequently used in the first millennium BCE. Unlike other communicable diseases in the ancient world, almost no records of concrete outbreaks of *šibṭu* exist. It is difficult to properly outline a word for

---

Neo-Assyrian period, besides at least one Middle Babylonian lexical entry (eSAD Š: *šabbiṭu*). For *šibṭu* as "sceptre" and "(beating-)stick", see also Kinnier Wilson 1956: 145.

63 RIMA 2: 193–194 Ashurnasirpal II A.0.101.1 col. i 4: . . . *na-din* GIŠ.GIDRU *u* EŠ.BAR *ana nap-ḫar* DÙ URU.URU . . ., the translation is as follows: "(Ninurta) the one who gives *sceptre* and (powers of) decision to all cities". Repeated in RIMA 2: 229 Ashurnasirpal II A.0.101.3 lines 7–8.

communal disaster, such as an epidemic, without a number of different case-studies or descriptions of symptomology. It is possible that *šibṭu* was conceptualized as something foreign, afflicting from outside everyday society. It could affect all spheres of society, from the individual, household, city and state, to the entire cosmos. Because the civilian population and professional healers only had a limited arsenal of therapeutic strategies available, the most common response to the dread induced by *šibṭu*, as a largescale catastrophe in society, remained prophylactic measures to keep the affliction at bay before it hit or to make it pass by once present. It remains unclear if the word was used interchangeably with other similar terms, such as *mūtānu*.

The word itself was derived from the verbal root *šabāṭu*, recording a sweeping motion when hitting someone, and *šibṭu* held violent connotations. The word held a close relation to the war and plague god Erra, particularly through this deity's cataclysmic actions in PEI. At least by the 1st millennium BCE, the verbal root became connected with the idea of a ruler's staff, used to administer judgement. It may therefore not have been accidental that *šipṭu* shared a relationship with the term *šipṭu* "judgement, punishment" through PEI. The callous rampage and mindless slaughter of the deity Erra encapsulated the nuances inherent in *šibṭu*, namely as a reference to a catastrophic event associated with war, slaughter, famine, and disease. Because the term may have been used for various widespread catastrophic events, potentially leading to sickness and death, researcher should be aware that a simple translation as "epidemic" or "plague" may not encapsulate all the nuances of *šibṭu* and it must be translated according to context.

Bibliography

Al-Rawi and Black 1989 = F. N. H. Al-Rawi and J. A. Black, 'The Second tablet of "Išum and Erra"', *Iraq* 51, 111–122

Ambos and Krauskopf 2010 = C. Ambos and I. Krauskopf, 'The Curved Staff in the Ancient Near East as a Predecessor of the Etruscan lituus', in: *Material Aspects of Etruscan Religion. Proceedings of the International Colloquium Leiden, May 29 and 30, 2008*, ed. L. B. van der Meer, BABESCH Annual Papers on Mediterranean Archaeology, Supplement 16 (Leuven, Paris, and Walpole: Peeters), 127–153

Arbøll 2018 = T. P. Arbøll, 'Tracing Mesopotamian Medical Knowledge: A Study of *maškadu-* and Related Illnesses', in: *Sources of Evil. Studies in Mesopotamian Exorcistic Lore*, ed. G. van Buylaere, M. Luukko, D. Schwemer and A. Mertens-Wagschal, Ancient Magic and Divination 15 (Leiden and Boston: Brill), 261–284

Arbøll 2021a = T. P. Arbøll, *Medicine in Ancient Assur: A Microhistorical Study of the Neo-Assyrian Healer Kiṣir-Aššur*, Ancient Magic and Divination 18 (Leiden and Boston: Brill)

Arbøll 2021b = T. P. Arbøll, 'Were People in Ancient Mesopotamia Aware of Zoonoses?', in: *Eskiçağda Salgın ve Hastalıklar*, ed. Ö. S. Gavaz and G. M. Ṣahin (Istanbul: Yayına Hazırlayanlar), 23–50

Arbøll 2023 = T. P. Arbøll, *The Cuneiform Texts from the Danish Excavations of Ḥamā in Syria (1931–1938): Letters, Administrative Documents, Scholarly Texts, Inscriptions, and Seals*, Scientia Danica. Series H, Humanistica 4 vol. 11 (Copenhagen: The Royal Danish Academy of Sciences and Letters)

Arbøll 2024 = T. P. Arbøll, 'Revisiting Epidemics in Cuneiform Sources: Ancient Attestations, Approaches, and Innovations', in: *Plague in Antiquity*, ed. *A. Jamieson, C. Tully, and L. Hitchcock*, Ancient Near Eastern Studies Supplement Series (Leuven, Paris, and Walpole: Peeters), 13–33

Bodel and Olyan 2008 = J. Bodel and S. M. Olyan, *Household and Family Religion in Antiquity* (Malden, Oxford, and Victoria: Blackwell Publishing)

Bottéro 1985 = J. Bottéro, *Mythes et Rites de Babylone* (Genève and Paris: Slatkine – Champion)

Böck 2014 = B. Böck, *The Healing Goddess Gula: Towards an Understanding of Ancient Babylonian Medicine*, Culture and History of the Ancient Near East 67 (Leiden and Boston: Brill)

Bramanti 2017 = A. Bramanti, 'The Scepter (ĜIDRU) in Early Mesopotamian Written Sources', *Kaskal* 14, 121–152

Cagni 1969 = L. Cagni, *L'Epopea di Erra*, Studi Semitici 34 (Rome: Instituto di Studi del Vicino Oriente)

Cagni 1970 = L. Cagni, *Das Erra-Epos. Keilschrifttext*, Studia Pohl 5 (Rome: Pontificium Institutum Biblicum)

Cagni 1977 = L. Cagni, *The Poem of Erra*, Sources of the Ancient Near East 1 (Malibu: Undena Publications)

Charpin 2006 = D. Charpin, 'G. Frame (éd.), *From the Upper Sea to the Lower Sea*' [Review], *Revue d'Assyriologie et d'archéologie orientale* 100, 180–182

Cooley 2008 = J. L. Cooley, '"I Want to Dim the Brilliance of Šulpae!" Mesopotamian Celestial Divination and the Poem of "Erra and Išum"', *Iraq* 70, 179–188

van Dijk 1962 = J. van Dijk, 'Die Inschriftenfunde', in: *Vorläufiger Bericht über die von dem Deutschen Archäologischen Institut und der Deutschen Orient-Gesellschaft aus Mitteln der Deutschen Forschungsgemeinschaft unternommenen Ausgrabungen in Uruk-Warka 18*, H. J. Lenzen, Abhandlungen der Deutschen Orient-Gesellschaft 7 (Berlin: Gebr. Mann), 39–62 and pl. 27

Dušek and Mynářová 2016 = J. Dušek and J. Mynářová, 'Tell Fekheriye Inscription: A Process of Authority on the Edge of the Assyrian Empire', in: *The Process of Authority. The Dynamics in Transmission and Reception of Canonical Texts*, ed. J. Dušek and J. Roskovec, Deuterocanonical and Cognate Literature Studies 27 (Berlin and Boston: De Gruyter), 9–40

Edzard 1976–80 = D. O. Edzard, 'Irra (Erra)', in: *Reallexikon der Assyriologie und Vorderasiatischen Archäologie. Fünfter Band. Ia . . . – Kizzuwatna*, ed. D. O. Edzard (Berlin and New York: Walter de Gruyter), 166–170

Farber 2004 = W. Farber, 'How to Marry a Disease: Epidemics, Contagion, and a Magic Ritual Against the "Hand of the Ghost"', in: *Magic and Rationality in Ancient Near Eastern and Graeco- Roman Medicine*, ed. H. F. J. Horstmanshoff and M. Stol (Leiden and Boston: Brill), 117–132

Farber 2008 = W. Farber, 'Die einleitende Episode des Erra-Epos', *Altorientalische Forschungen* 35, 262–267

Feder 2022 = Y. Feder, *Purity and Pollution in the Hebrew Bible. From Embodied Experience to Moral Metaphor* (Cambridge, New York, Port Melbourne, New Delhi, and Singapore: Cambridge University Press)

Fincke 2000 = J. Fincke, *Augenleiden nach keilschriftlichen Quellen: Untersuchungen zur altorientalischen Medizin*, Würzburger medizinhistorische Forschungen 70 (Würzburg: Königshausen & Neumann)

Fleming 2008 = D. E. Fleming, 'The Integration of Household and Community Religion in Ancient Syria', in: *Household and Family Religion in Antiquity*, ed. J. Bodel and S. M. Olyan (Malden, Oxford, and Victoria: Blackwell Publishing), 37–59

Foster 2005 = B. Foster, *Before the Muses: An Anthology of Akkadian Literature* [Third edition] (Bethesda: CDL Press)

Franke 2014 = S. Franke, 'Der Zorn Marduks, Erras und Sanheribs zu Dateierung und Funktion von "Erra und Išum"', in: *Krieg und Frieden im Alten Vorderasien. 52e Rencontre Assyriologique Internationale Münster, 17.–21. Juli 2006*, ed. H. Neumann, R. Dittmann, S. Paulus, G. Neumann, and A. Schuster-Brandis, Alter Orient und Altes testament 401 (Münster: Ugarit-Verlag), 315–327

Gelb 1980 = I. J. Gelb, *Computer-aided Analysis of Amorite*, Assyriological Studies 21 (Chicago: The Oriental Institute of the University of Chicago)

Geller 2016 = M. J. Geller, *Healing Magic and Evil Demons: Canonical Udug-hul Incantations*, Die babylonisch-assyrische Medizin in Texten und Untersuchungen 8 (Boston and Berlin: De Gruyter)

Geller 2018 = M. J. Geller, 'The Exorcist's Manual (KAR 44)' in *Assyrian and Babylonian Scholarly Text Catalogues*, ed. U. Steinert, Die babylonisch-assyrische Medizin in Texten und Untersuchungen 9 (Boston and Berlin: De Gruyter), 292–312

George 2003 = A. R. George, *The Babylonian Gilgamesh Epic: Introduction, Critical Edition and Cuneiform Texts, Volume I–II* (Oxford: Oxford University Press)

George 2013 = A. R. George, 'The Poem of Erra and Ishum: A Babylonian Poet's View of War', in: *Warfare and Poetry in the Middle East*, ed. H. Kennedy (London and New York: Bloomsbury Publishing), 39–71.

Goetze 1939 = A. Geotze, 'Cuneiform Inscriptions from Tarsus', *Journal of the American Oriental Society* 59/1, 1–16

Gössmann 1955 = P. F. Gössmann, *Das Era-Epos* (Würzburg: Augustinus-Verlag)

Heeßel 2009–10 = N. P. Heeßel, 'Seuche', in: *Reallexikon der Assyriologie und Vorderasiatischen Archäologie. Band 12. Samuha–Sililitu*, ed. M. P. Streck (Berlin: De Gruyter), 405–406

Heeßel 2014 = N. P. Heeßel, 'Amulette und "Amulettform": Zum Zusammenhand von Form, Funktion und Text von Amuletten im Alten Mesopotamien', in: *Erscheinungsformen und Handhabungen heiliger Schriften*, ed. J. F. Quack and D. C. Luft, Materielle Textkulturen 5 (Berlin, München, and Boston: De Gruyter), 53–77

Helle 2018 = S. Helle, 'The Role of Authors in the "Uruk List of Kings and Sages": Canonization and Cultural Contact', *Journal of Near Eastern Studies* 77/2, 219–234

Hruška 1973 = B. Hruška, 'Einige Überlegungen zum Erraepos', *Bibliotheca Orientalis* 30, 3–7

Jacobsen 1939 = T. Jacobsen, *The Sumerian King List*, Assyriological Studies 11 (Chicago: The University of Chicago Press)

Jiménez 2017 = E. Jiménez, *The Babylonian Disputation Poems*, Culture and History of the Ancient Near East 87 (Leiden and Boston: Brill)

Jiménez 2018 = E. Jiménez, 'Highway to Hell: The Winds as Cosmic Conveyors in Mesopotamian Incantation Texts', in: *Sources of Evil. Studies in Mesopotamian Exorcistic Lore*, ed. G. van Buylaere, M. Luukko, D. Schwemer and A. Mertens-Wagschal, Ancient Magic and Divination 15 (Leiden and Boston: Brill), 316–350

Joannès 2022 = F. Joannès, '"Lorsqu'une épizootie s'y est déclarée . . ." (*Šibṭu kī ina libbi iššaknu*)', *Journal des Médecines Cunéiformes* 39, 1–9

Kinnier Wilson 1956 = J. V. Kinnier Wilson, 'Two Medical Texts from Nimrud', *Iraq* 18/2, 130–146

Kleber 2012 = K. Kleber, 'Famine in Babylonia. A Microhistorical approach to an agricultural crisis in 528–526 BC', *Zeitschrift für Assyriologie* 102, 219–244

Koch-Westenholz 1995 = U. S. Koch-Westenholz, *Mesopotamian Astrology: An Introduction to Babylonian and Assyrian Celestial Divination*, CNI Publications 19 (Copenhagen: Museum Tusculanum Press)

Kozuh 2014 = M. Kozuh, *The Sacrificial Economy. Assessors, Contractors, and Thieves in the Management of Sacrificial Sheep at the Eanna Temple of Uruk (ca. 625–520 B.C.)*, Explorations in Ancient Near Eastern Civilizations 2 (Winona Lake: Eisenbrauns)

Krahmalkov 2000 = C. R. Krahmalkov, *Phoenician-Punic Dictionary*, Studia Phoenicia 15 (Leuven: Peeters)

Kvanvig 2011 = H. S. Kvanvig, *Primeval History: Babylonian, Biblical, and Enochic*, Supplements to the Journal for the Study of Judaism 149 (Leiden and Boston: Brill)

Köcher 1965 = F. Köcher, 'Urruru, "(am Feuer) dörren"', in: *Studies in Honor of Benno Landsberger on His Seventy-fifth Birthday April 21, 1965*, ed. H. G. Güterbock and T. Jacobsen, Assyriological Studies 1 (Chicago: The University of Chicago Press), 323–325

Lambert 1970 = W. G. Lambert, 'Fire Incantations', *Archiv für Orientforschung* 23, 39–45 and pls. 1–9

Lambert 1973 = W. G. Lambert, 'Studies in Nergal' [Review of von Weiher 1971], *Bibliotheca Orientalis* 30, 355–363

Lambert 2007 = W. G. Lambert, *Babylonian Oracle Questions*, Mesopotamian Civilizations 13 (Winona Lake: Eisenbrauns)

Leichty and Walker 2004 = E. Leichty and C. B. F. Walker, 'Three Babylonian Chronicle and Scientific Texts', in: *From the Upper Sea to the Lower Sea. Studies on the History of Assyria and Babylonia in Honour of A.K. Grayson*, Publications de l' Institut Historique et Archeologique Néerlandais de Stanboul 101 (Leiden: Nederlands Instituut voor het Nabije Oosten), 203–212

Lewis 2008 = T. J. Lewis, 'Family, Household, and Local Religion at Late Bronze Age Ugarit', in: *Household and Family Religion in Antiquity*, ed. J. Bodel and S. M. Olyan (Malden, Oxford, and Victoria: Blackwell Publishing), 60–88

Lipiński 1994 = E. Lipiński, *Studies in Aramaic Inscriptions and Onomastics II*, Orientalia Lovaniensia Analecta 58 (Leuven: Peeters)

Lipiński 2000 = E. Lipiński, *The Aramaeans. Their Ancient History, Culture, Religion*, Orientalia Lovaniensia Analecta 100 (Leuven, Paris, and Sterling: Peeters)

Machinist 1981 = P. Machinist, 'The Poem of Erra. By Luigi Cagni' [Review], *Journal of the American Oriental Society* 101, 401–403

Machinist and Sasson 1983 = P. Machinist and J. M. Sasson, 'Rest and Violence in the Poem of Erra', *Journal of the American Oriental Society* 103, 221–226

Maul 1994 = S. M. Maul, *Zukunftsbewältigung: Eine Untersuchung altorientalischen Denkens anhand der babylonisch-assyrischen Löserituale (Namburbi)*, Baghdader Forschungen 18 (Mainz: Verlag Philipp von Zabern)

Nakata 1979 = I. Nakata, 'A Few Remarks on the Study of Deities – a Review Article on J. J. M. Roberts, *The Earliest Semitic Pantheon.* Baltimore-London 1972' [Review], *Acta Sumerologica* 1, 63–68

Noegel 2011 = S. B. Noegel, '"Wordplay" in the Song of Erra', in: *Strings and Threads. A Celebration of the Work of Anne Draffkorn Kilmer*, ed. W. Heimpel and G. Frantz-Szabó (Winona Lake: Eisenbrauns), 161–193 del Olmo Lete and Sanmartín 2003 = G. del Olmo Lete and J. Sanmartín, *A Dictionary of the Ugaritic Language in the Alphabetic Tradition* [Translated by W.G.E. Watson], Handbuch der Orientalistik 67 (Leiden and Boston: Brill)

Panayotov 2018 = S. V. Panayotov, 'Magico-medical Plants and Incantations on Assyrian House Amulets', in: *Sources of Evil. Studies in Mesopotamian Exorcistic Lore*, ed. G. van Buylaere, M. Luukko, D. Schwemer, and A. Mertens-Wagschal, Ancient Magic and Divination 15 (Leiden and Boston: Brill), 192–222

Radner 2005 = K. Radner, *Die Macht des Namens. Altorientalische Strategien zur Selbsterhaltung*, SANTAG 8 (Wiesbaden: Harrassowitz)

Al-Rawi and George 1991–92 = F. N. H. Al-Rawi and A. R. George, 'Enūma Anu Enlil XIV and Other Early Astronomical Tablets', *Archiv für Orientforschung* 38–39, 52–73

Reiner 1958 = E. Reiner, *Šurpu: A Collection of Sumerian and Akkadian Incantations*, Archiv für Orientforschung Beiheft 11 (Osnabrück: Biblio Verlag)

Reiner 1960 = E. Reiner, 'Plague Amulets and House Blessings', *Journal of Near Eastern Studies* 19/2, 149–155

Roberts 1971 = J. J. M. Roberts, 'Erra: Scorched Earth', *Journal of Cuneiform Studies* 24, 11–16

Salin 2015 = S. Salin, 'When Disease "Touches", "Hits", or "Seizes" in Assyro-Babylonian Medicine', *Kaskal* 12, 319–336

San Nicolò 1954 = M. San Nicolò, 'Materialien zur Viehwirtschaft in den neubabylonischen Tempeln. IV', *Orientalia* 23, 351–382

Scheidel 2017 = W. Scheidel, *The Great Leveler. Violence and the History of Inequality from the Stone Age to the Twenty-First Century* (Princeton and Oxford: Princeton University Press)

Schramm 2008 = W. Schramm, *Ein Compendium sumerisch-akkadischer Beschwörungen*, Göttinger Beiträge zum Alten Orient Band 2 (Göttingen: Universitätsverlag Göttingen)

Schramm unpublished = W. Schramm, *Sumerisch-Akkadische Beschwörungstexte* [Unpublished manuscript, the title written as printed] (Göttingen)

Schuster-Brandis 2008 = A. Schuster-Brandis, *Steine als Schutz- und Heilmittel*, Alter Orient und Altes Testament 46 (Münster: Ugarit-Verlag)

Scurlock and Andersen 2005 = J. A. Scurlock and B. R. Andersen, *Diagnoses in Assyrian and Babylonian Medicine: Ancient Sources, Translations, and Modern Medical Analyses* (Urbana and Chicago: University of Illinois Press)

Steinkeller 2004 = P. Steinkeller, 'Studies in Third Millennium Paleography, 4: Sign KIŠ', *Zeitschrift für Assyriologie* 94, 175–185

Stol 1993 = M. Stol, *Epilepsy in Babylonia*, Cuneiform Monographs 2 (Groningen: Styx Publications)

Tarasewicz 2017 = R. Tarasewicz, 'More about the Crisis in Uruk', in: *Fortune and Misfortune in the Ancient Near East. Proceedings of the 60th Rencontre Assyriologique Internationale at Warsaw 21–25 July 2014*, ed. O. Drewnowska and M. Sandowicz (Winona Lake: Eisenbrauns), 347–355

Taylor 2017 = K. Taylor, *The Erra Song: A Religious, Literary, and Comparative Analysis* [PhD dissertation, Harvard University] (Cambridge)

Thureau-Dangin 1912 = F. Thureau-Dangin, *Une Relation de la huitième Campagne de Sargon (714 av. J.-C.)* (Paris: Librairie Paul Geuthner)

van der Toorn 2008 = K. van der Toorn, 'Family Religion in Second Millennium West Asia (Mesopotamia, Emar, Nuzi)', in: *Household and Family Religion in Antiquity*, ed. J. Bodel and S. M. Olyan (Malden, Oxford, and Victoria: Blackwell Publishing), 20–36

Waerzeggers 2015 = C. Waerzeggers, 'The Neo-Babylonian chronicle about Sabium and Apil-Sîn: a copy of the text (BM 29440)', *NABU* 2015/54, 85

Wasserman 2012 = N. Wasserman, '*Maškadum* and Other Zoonotic Diseases in Medical and Literary Akkadian Sources', *Bibliotheca Orientalis* 69, 426–436

von Weiher 1971 = E. von Weiher, *Der babylonische Gott Nergal*, Alter Orient und Altes Testament 11 (Neukirchen-Vluyn: Verlag Butzon & Bercker Kevelaer and Neukirchener Verlag)

Westenholz 1997 = J. G. Westenholz, *Legends of the Kings of Agade*, Mesopotamian Civilizations 7 (Winona Lake: Eisenbrauns)

Wiggermann 1992 = F. A. M. Wiggermann, *Mesopotamian Protective Spirits: The Ritual Texts*, Cuneiform Monographs 1 (Groningen: Styx & PP Publications)

Wiggermann 1999 = F. A. M. Wiggermann, 'Nergal. A. Philologisch', in: *Reallexikon der Assyriologie und Vorderasiatischen Archäologie. Band 9 3./4. Lieferung. Nanše–^{d}NIM.NIM*, ed. D. O. Edzard (Berlin and New York: De Gruyter), 215–223

Wisnom 2019 = S. Wisnom, *Weapons of Words: Intertextual Competition in Babylonian Poetry*, Culture and History of the Ancient Near East 106 (Leiden and Boston: Brill)

Wunsch 2003 = C. Wunsch, *Urkunden zum Ehe-, Vermögens- und Erbrecht aus verschiedenen neubabylonischen Archiven*, Babylonische Archive 2 (Dresden: Islet)

Indices

Texts Cited

 | https://doi.org/10.1515/9783112238622-009

Sumerian and Akkadian Terms Discussed

Deities Discussed

Ancient People Discussed

Places Discussed, Ancient and Modern

General Index

www.ingramcontent.com/pod-product-compliance
Lightning Source LLC
Jackson TN
JSHW061514070526
102001JS00005B/11
9783112238615